MODULATING GENE EXPRESSION - ABRIDGING THE RNAI AND CRISPR-CAS9 TECHNOLOGIES

Edited by **Aditi Singh**
and **Mohammad W. Khan**

Modulating Gene Expression - Abridging the RNAi and CRISPR-Cas9 Technologies
http://dx.doi.org/10.5772/intechopen.75144
Edited by Aditi Singh and Mohammad W. Khan

Contributors

Lingwen Zeng, Shi-Lin Cao, Omar Mukama, Dong-Hai Lin, Xuewen Lu, Amal Qattan, Moises Zotti, Deise Cagliari, Ericmar Avila Dos Santos, Naymã Dias, Guy Smagghe, Saurav Mallik, Tapas Bhadra, Namrata Tomar, Ayan Mukherji, Ujjwal Maulik, Manuel Sanchez-Martin, Ignacio Garcia-Tuñon, Takeshi Yasuda, Katsushi Tajima, Aditi Singh

Notice

First published in London, United Kingdom, 2019 by IntechOpen
IntechOpen is the global imprint of INTECHOPEN LIMITED, registered in England and Wales, registration number: 11086078, The Shard, 25th floor, 32 London Bridge Street
London, SE19SG – United Kingdom
Printed in Croatia

British Library Cataloguing-in-Publication Data
A catalogue record for this book is available from the British Library

Additional hard and PDF copies can be obtained from orders@intechopen.com

Modulating Gene Expression - Abridging the RNAi and CRISPR-Cas9 Technologies, Edited by Aditi Singh and Mohammad W. Khan

p. cm.

Print ISBN 978-1-83880-696-5
Online ISBN 978-1-83880-697-2
eBook (PDF) ISBN 978-1-83880-698-9

For EU product safety concerns:
IN TECH d.o.o., Prolaz Marije Krucifikse Kozulić 3, 51000 Rijeka, Croatia,
info@intechopen.com or visit our website at intechopen.com.

Meet the editors

Aditi Singh is a research enthusiast, working as an application scientist in a biotechnology company. She has a PhD degree in molecular-cell biology from the University of Heidelberg in Germany and worked as a postdoctoral scholar at the University of California San Diego, USA. Aditi has more than nine years of experience in the field of molecular and cell biology, where she has been involved in various R&D projects and technical support. Her research interests are cell biology, RNA biology, gene editing, and infectious diseases.

Mohammad W. Khan is a research enthusiast, working as an application scientist in a biotechnology company. He has a PhD degree from the University of Heidelberg in Germany and a DVM degree from Maharashtra Animal and Fishery Sciences University, Nagpur, India. He also worked as a postdoctoral scholar at San Diego State University, USA.
Dr Khan has more than 15 years of experience in the field of molecular and cell biology, where he has been involved in various R&D projects and technical support. He has authored and reviewed several research articles and has also served as guest editor for several high-impact journals.
His research interests are protein biology, RNA biology, cancer research, immunology, genomics, gene editing, and infectious diseases.

Contents

Preface

RNA interference (RNAi) is a widely used technology for gene silencing and has become a key tool in a myriad of research and lead discoveries. In recent years, the mechanism of RNAi agents has been well investigated, and the technique has been optimized for better effectiveness and safety. In the last few decades, advances in RNAi technology and the potential for leveraging RNAi for sequence-specific gene silencing have put it at the forefront for developing effective therapeutics against an array of diseases. siRNAs have been successfully used in a variety of experimental settings both in vivo and in vitro, thereby permitting long-lasting silencing of genes of interest.

Alongside this, the clustered regularly interspaced short palindromic repeats (CRISPR)-associated Cas9/gRNA system is a fairly recent, novel, targeted, genome-editing technique derived from the bacterial immune system. Recent advances in gene-editing research and technologies have enabled the CRISPR-Cas9 system to become a popular tool for sequence-specific gene editing to correct and modify eukaryotic systems. The technology allows targeted knock-ins and knocks-outs of any gene within the genome. DNA mutations ranging from a single base pair to large deletions in both in vitro and in vivo model systems have been accomplished, thereby revolutionizing the molecular biology world of science.

In this book, we will focus on the mechanisms, applications, regulations (their pros and cons), and various ways in which RNAi-based methods and CRIPSR-Cas9 technology have stimulated the modulation of gene expression, thereby making them a promising therapeutic tool to treat and prevent complex diseases and disorders.

Aditi Singh and Mohammad W. Khan
Independent scientists, USA

Section 1

Introduction

Chapter 1

Introductory Chapter: Modulating Gene Expression - Abridging the RNAi and CRISPR-Cas9 Technologies

Aditi Singh

Additional information is available at the end of the chapter

http://dx.doi.org/10.5772/intechopen.84229

1. Gene-silencing technologies over the years

Silencing a gene by deleting it, knocking it down, or simply disabling its function has proven to be a promising tool for understanding the function of the gene and to enable lead optimization during drug development process. In recent times, the two commonly used gene modification methods that have been heavily explored are RNA interference (RNAi) and the revolutionary CRISPR/Cas9 system.

RNA interference (RNAi) is a widely used technology for gene-silencing and has become a critical tool for repression of gene expression which is effectively utilized in various researches. Of late, the mechanism of RNA interference has been well investigated, and undergone various levels of optimization for improving its effectiveness and efficiency.

The clustered regularly interspaced short palindromic repeats (CRISPR)-associated Cas9/gRNA system on the other hand, is a unique, targeted genome-modification technique derived from prokaryotic immune system. The cutting edge research and technology advancements in recent years have enabled the CRISPR-Cas9 system to become a popular tool for introducing heritable, precised, insertions and deletions in the eukaryotic genome.

1.1. Mechanism of the two prominent gene-silencing technologies

The two technologies, however, vastly differ in their mode of action. RNAi uses small interfering RNA molecules to deplete target mRNAs by triggering their degradation and silencing the gene. In RNAi, short, double-stranded RNA molecules, called small interfering RNAs (siRNAs), bind to messenger RNAs (mRNAs) that bear complementary sequences, and blocks the translation of protein encoded by the mRNA. On the other hand, CRISPR/Cas9 system also known as "molecular scissors" can introduce precise and targeted change within the genome.

The technique involves designing specific "single guide RNAs" (sgRNAs) that recognize specific sequences in the genome known as PAM sites. Once the Cas9 proteins along with this sgRNA are introduced into the cells, small deletions occur adjacent to the PAM site via double-stranded DNA breaks. The CRISPR/Cas9 system has been adapted to inhibit the expression of single or multiple genetic loci wherein it cleaves specific DNA sequences, thereby rendering the gene nonfunctional.

1.2. Abridging the two prominent gene-silencing technologies

Although mechanistically different, the two techniques may complement one another very well. Genes can be knocked down with RNA interference (RNAi) or knocked out with CRISPR-Cas9; when used together, they facilitate the discovery and validation of scientific findings. Researchers can do a whole genome RNAi library screen now by using synthetic siRNAs, and then validate each target by designing specific sgRNAs and utilizing the CRISPR-Cas9 technology.

2. Future of these gene-silencing technologies

While the RNAi technique ruled the tailoring of eukaryotic gene expression in the last two decades, the CRISPR/Cas9 system is fairly pretty recent and therefore requires much more exploration and optimization. The superiority of the CRISPR/Cas9 system in effectiveness and efficiency, along with its vast popularity among research community certainly raises the question if in coming years the RNAi technology is going to be obsolete. Application wise, the CRISPR/Cas9 technology truly has the potential to outweigh the RNAi technology, but there is a long road ahead before we can freely make permanent edits to human DNA.

Author details

Aditi Singh

Address all correspondence to: aditi.ucsd@gmail.com

Independent Scientist, USA

Section 2

Gene Silencing Applications

Chapter 2

CRISPR-ERA for Switching Off (Onco) Genes

Ignacio García-Tuñon, Elena Vuelta,
Sandra Pérez-Ramos, Jesús M Hernández-Rivas,
Lucía Méndez, María Herrero and
Manuel Sanchez-Martin

Additional information is available at the end of the chapter

http://dx.doi.org/10.5772/intechopen.80245

Abstract

Genome-editing nucleases like the popular CRISPR/Cas9 enable the generation of knockout cell lines and null zygotes by inducing site-specific double-stranded breaks (DSBs) within a genome. In most cases, when a DNA template is not present, the DSB is repaired by nonhomologous end joining (NHEJ), resulting in small nucleotide insertions or deletions that can be used to construct knockout alleles. However, for several reasons, these mutations do not produce the desired null result in all cases, instead generating a similar protein with functional activity. This undesirable effect could limit the therapeutic efficiency of gene therapy strategies focused on abrogating oncogene expression by CRISPR/Cas9 and should be taken into account. This chapter reviews the irruption of CRISPR technology for gene silencing and its application in gene therapy.

Keywords: gene therapy, knockout, null allele, oncogene silencing, CRISPR technology, gene suppression

1. Gene suppression therapies in cancer: an overview

Gene therapy, which was initially developed for the treatment of genetic (primarily monogenic) diseases, has mainly focused on cancer therapy, so that more than 65% of all gene therapy trials worldwide (**Figure 1**) are aimed at the treatment of solid and hematological malignancies [1]. As a consequence, cancer gene therapy is a predominant field of basic research, as well as of clinical activities (**Table 1**) [2].

Various strategies at different molecular levels (**Figure 2**) have been employed to treat malignant diseases in recent decades, such as specific drug inhibitors acting at the protein level,

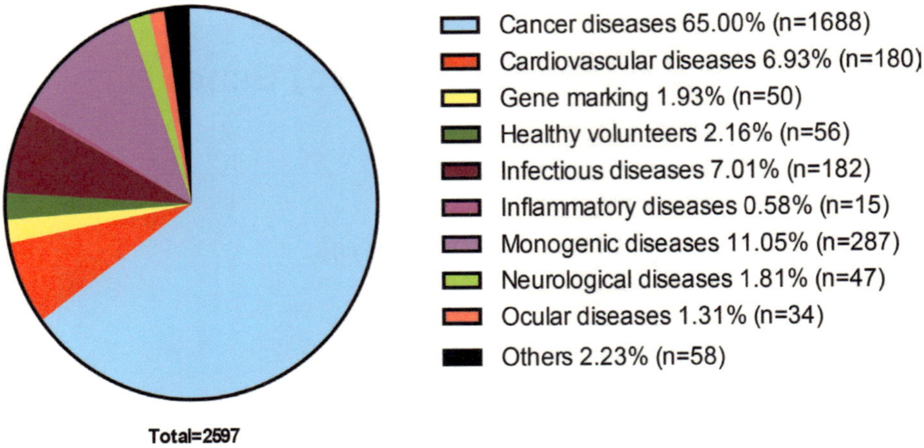

Figure 1. Gene therapy trials worldwide.

Indications	Gene therapy clinical trials	
	Number	%
Cancer diseases	1688	65.0
Cardiovascular diseases	180	6.9
Gene marking	50	1.9
Healthy volunteers	56	2.2
Infectious diseases	182	7.0
Inflammatory diseases	15	0.6
Monogenic diseases	287	11.1
Neurological diseases	47	1.8
Ocular diseases	34	1.3
Others	58	2.2

Table 1. Gene therapy trials worldwide.

gene suppression therapies at the mRNA level, and genome-editing nucleases at the DNA level [3].

The ability of several drugs to inhibit the activity of a targeted oncoprotein has been exploited as a therapeutic approach for a variety of malignancies, the best example being imatinib mesylate, a tyrosine-kinase inhibitor (TKI) indicated for the first-line treatment of chronic myeloid leukemia (CML). The advent of imatinib mesylate at the end of the twentieth century has revolutionized CML prognosis, yielding an overall survival (OS) rate of 88% after 5 years, whereas previous nonspecific treatments produced an OS rate of only 57% [4]. Unfortunately, despite the increased efficacy and better clinical responses, many patients receiving targeted drugs have a poor initial response, develop resistance, or undergo relapse after initial success. Except for a subgroup of patients who achieve a deep and sustained molecular response, TKI

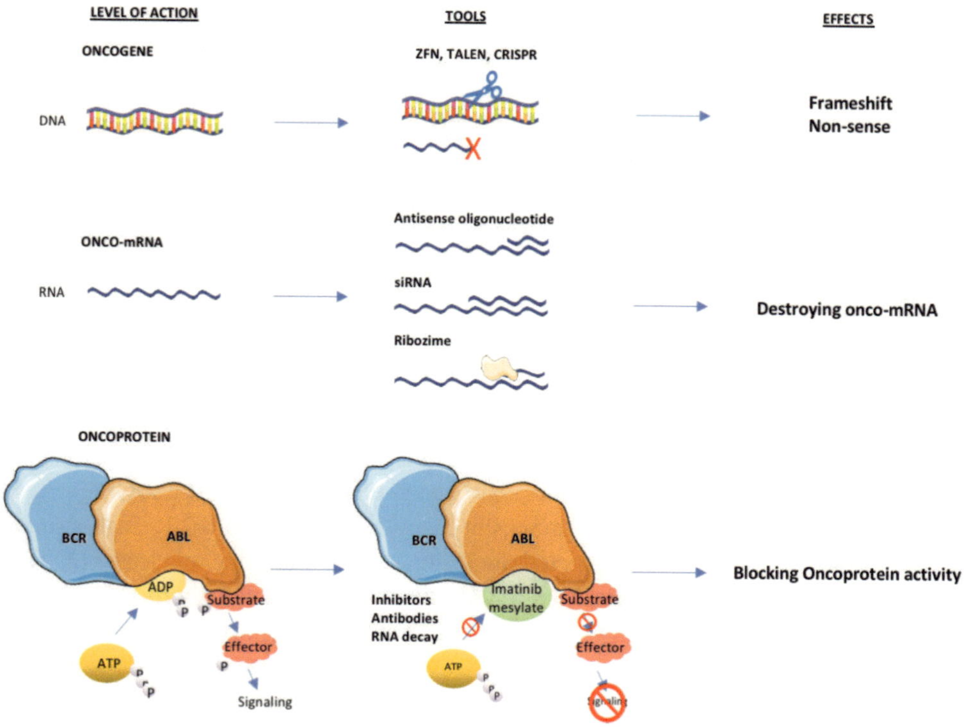

Figure 2. Different strategies to block oncogene effects.

therapies would need to be continued indefinitely because TKIs do not completely eliminate the leukemia stem cells (LSCs), but they remain even during effective TKI treatment [5].

An alternative oncoprotein inhibition approach emerges from the ability of some small RNAs to fold into three-dimensional structures that can then bind to proteins and thereby inhibit them in a manner similar to protein antagonists [6]. This is the logic behind the use of RNA "decoys" or RNA aptamers. Recent preclinical and clinical data support the potential activity of a 45-nucleotide-long RNA aptamer (NOX-A12) that specifically antagonizes the CXC chemokine ligand 12/stromal cell-derived factor-1 (CXCL 12/SDF-1), which is a regulatory chemokine essential for the migration of leukemic stem cells into the bone marrow [6]. This inhibition of the binding of SDF-1 to its receptors can prompt the leukemic stem cells to re-enter the cell cycle and become vulnerable to chemotherapeutic attack.

Other gene suppression therapies focus on the intervention of gene transcription and translation, which are vital elements for cancer growth, spread, survival, and therapy resistance. Ribozymes, antisense oligodeoxynucleotides (AS-ODNs), and short-interfering RNAs (siRNAs) are an emerging class of targeted DNA-based pharmaceuticals. Ribozymes, a subset of catalytic RNAs, can be artificially synthesized and used to specifically suppress gene function. They can also be used to validate disease-related genes as potential targets for new therapeutic interventions. Their ability to cleave mRNA to prevent protein synthesis enables them to be applied in cancer and virology. Transcripts of genes of different function have been targeted by AS-ODN gene therapies such as c-myb, c-raf, c-fos, H-ras, Her2/neu, bcl-2, VEGF, and Ang-1. The use of AS-ODNs was shown to successfully inhibit gene expression in association with tumor growth inhibition, radiosensitization, or chemosensitization [7–9]. The use of siRNA technology provides another novel approach for targeted sequence-specific suppression of target gene expression. In this system, siRNA stability and proper delivery are key factors for successful application. *In vitro* and *in vivo* studies with siRNA targeting PKN3 mRNA have been successful at inhibiting tumor progression and metastasis in lung and mammary carcinoma models [10]. Nonetheless, inefficient/complete silencing and transient effects present major challenges to cancer gene therapy mediated by ribozymes, AS-ODNs, or siRNAs [2]. Other important challenges that need to be addressed for the successful translation of these approaches are their delivery to the site of action, the choice between direct delivery or the use of a vehicle, mass production at low cost, more clearly defined pharmacokinetics, and the ability to produce sustained long-term effects, immunogenicity, and toxicity (including inappropriate or excessive expression).

With the recent explosion of genome editing tools, including clustered, regularly interspaced short palindromic repeats and their nuclease-associated protein Cas9 (CRISPR/Cas9), the landscape of suppression techniques has dramatically changed. Although CRISPR/Cas9 is similar in action and efficacy to protein-based targeted nucleases, such as zinc finger nucleases (ZFNs) and transcription activator-like effector nucleases (TALENs) [11], the ease with which these reagents can be designed and tested through the construction of single-guide RNAs (sgRNAs) has made gene editing available to a wider variety of users and for a broader range of applications.

CRISPR/Cas9 works at the DNA level and has the advantage of providing permanent and full gene knockout, while AS-ODNs and siRNAs only silence genes transiently because they working at the mRNA level [12, 13]. CRISPR/Cas9 cuts DNA in a sequence-specific manner with the possibility of interrupting coding sequences, thereby making it possible to turn off cancer drivers in a way that was not previously feasible in humans [14, 15]. This notable application of permanent gene disruption is based on the cellular mechanisms involved in double-stranded break (DSB) repair.

2. CRISPR-Cas9 technology, DSBs, and gene interruption

The CRISPR/Cas9 system allows sequence-specific gene editing in many organisms and is currently the best tool for generating cell lines and animal models of human diseases. The main advantages of this technology are its simplicity, versatility, and efficiency compared with other gene-modifying technologies. CRISPR/Cas9 technology is usually used to introduce targeted DSBs in any biological system [16], and the only requirement for Cas9-mediated DNA recognition and cleavage is the presence of a short protospacer adjacent motif (PAM) immediately 3′ to the targeted DNA sequence [17] (**Figure 3**).

Following the creation of a DSB within the coding sequence of a gene, mechanisms of DNA repair can induce insertions and deletions (indels), resulting in frameshift or nonsense mutations [18]. Basically, the repair of DSBs involves four possible mechanisms (**Figure 4**). The first mechanism is standard nonhomologous end-joining (C-NHEJ). In this mechanism, the DSB is repaired by blunt-end ligation independently of sequence homology and requires DNA ligase IV action (**Figure 1A**). C-NHEJ can occur throughout the cell cycle but is dominant in G0/G1

http://dx.doi.org/10.5772/intechopen.80245

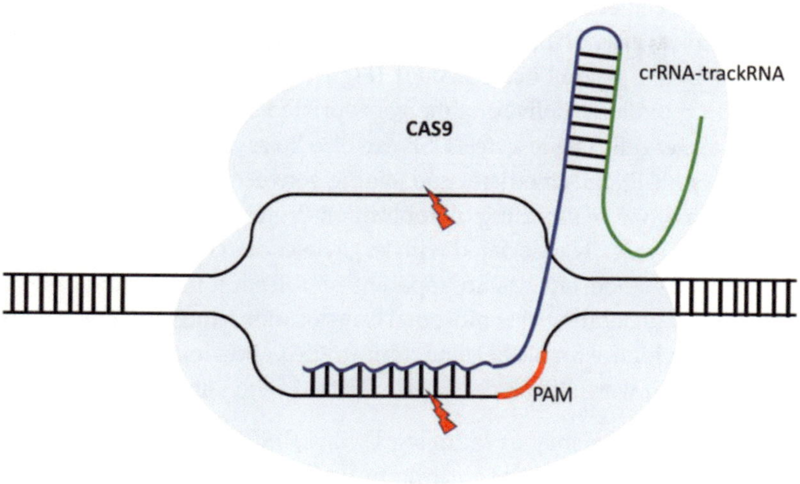

Figure 3. CRISPR/Cas9 ribonucleoprotein complex. Cas9 nuclease is driven to the target DNA sequence by an sgRNA molecule, composed by crRNA (blue) and trackRNA (green). The target sequence must be followed immediately by a protospacer adjacent motif sequence (PAM). After hybridization of 20 nt of the cRNA with the target sequence, the nuclease performs a double-stranded break 3 nt upstream of the PAM sequence.

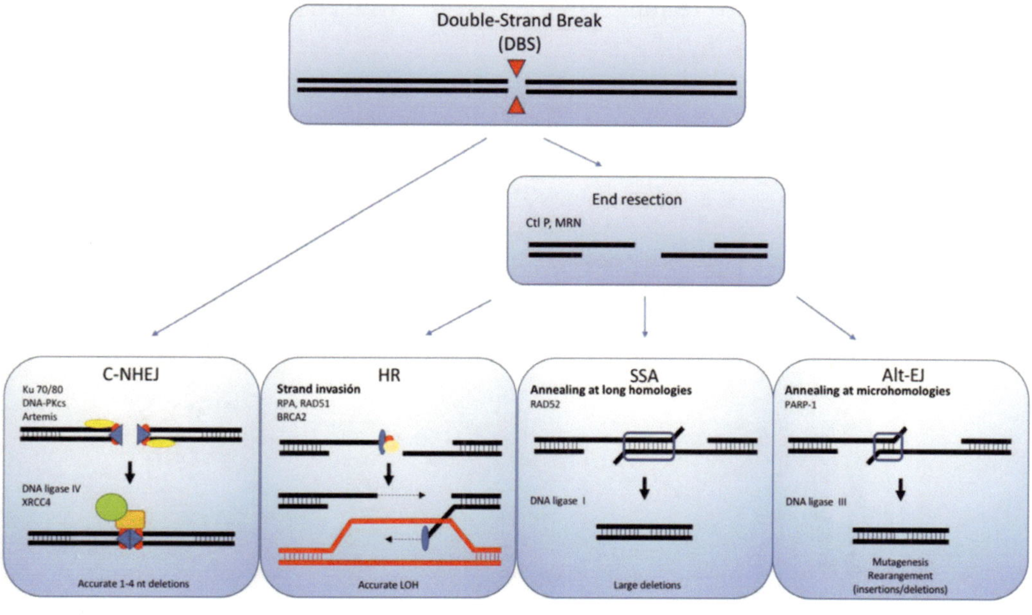

Figure 4. Approaches to repair DNA double-strand breaks. When DNA resection is blocked, C-NHEJ (classic nonhomologous end joining) is well established, whereas if the resection does occur, DNA damage is repaired by HR (homologous recombination), SSA (single-strand annealing) or alt-EJ (alternative end joining) [18].

and G2 and is associated with 1–4 bp deletions [19], which could produce frameshift mutations. Alternatively, the DSB end can be resected, leaving 3′ single-stranded DNA (ssDNA) overhangs. The resected DSB can be repaired by three possible mechanisms: homologous recombination (HR), single-strand annealing (SSA), and alternative end joining (alt-EJ). HR predominates in the mid-S and mid-G2 cell cycle phases, where the amount of DNA replication is highest and when the sister template is available [20]. HR uses a template for repair and so requires strand invasion mediated by the recombinase RAD51 (**Figure 4**) [21]. It may be possible to exploit this property to edit mutations, delivering the appropriate template joined to the CRISPR/Cas9 system inside the target cell. The resected DSB can also be repaired by mutagenic repair pathways, namely SSA or alt-EJ. SSA mediates end joining between interspersed nucleotide repeats in the genome and involves reannealing of Replication Protein A (RPA)-covered ssDNA by the RAD52 protein. SSA is typically associated with large deletions (**Figure 4**) [21]. The alt-EJ mechanism is not well understood but has an apparent predilection for joining DSBs on different chromosomes, thereby generating chromosomal translocations and mutagenic rearrangements (**Figure 4**) [22]. Early evidence for alt-EJ came from studies, showing that yeast and mammalian cells deficient in C-NHEJ were still able to repair DSBs via end joining [23].

As a consequence of its efficiency at inducing DSB, CRISPR/Cas9 technology has gained a reputation as the "gold standard" for creating null alleles in both *in vivo* and *in vitro*. These null alleles can arise from frameshift mutations, premature stop codons, and/or non-sense-mediated decay on the target gene, resulting in loss of function. Currently, CRISPR/Cas9 is extensively used to engineer gene knockouts, but due to the variable size of the NHEJ-induced indel, generating a full KO in one step is not always achieved. In fact, full KO generation requires off-frame mutations in both alleles, and this is a matter of probability because several mutations could preserve the reading frame (e.g., +3 or −3 mutations). This undesirable effect

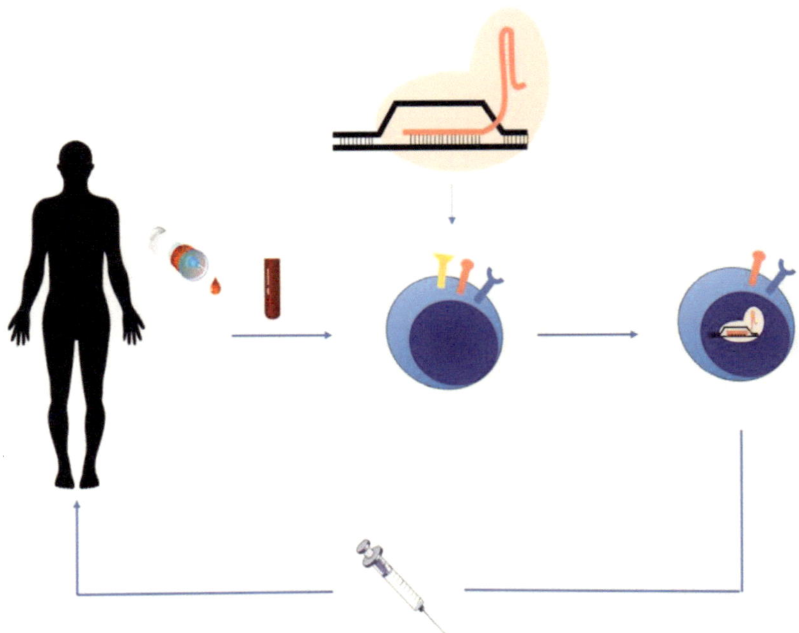

Figure 5. Experimental design of the first CRISPR/Cas9-edited cell injection in humans. Immune precursor cells were isolated from blood and *in vitro* CRISPR/Cas9 edited to eliminate PD-1 gene. Modified cells were then reinfused into the patient [25].

may be irrelevant in assays in which the knockout cell can be selected, or the null allele of the animal model can be segregated [24]. The first clinical trial using CRISPR for gene suppression and cancer therapy enrolled its first patient at Sichuan University's West China Hospital in Chengdu in 2016 [25]. In this study, the safety of PD-1 knockout CRISPR-engineered T cells *ex vivo* was evaluated when treating metastatic non–small cell lung cancer that had progressed after employing all standard treatments. Patients enrolled in the gene-editing trial provided peripheral blood lymphocytes, and PD-1 knockout of T-cells by CRISPR/Cas9 was performed *ex vivo*. In this trial, the edited lymphocytes were selected, expanded, and subsequently infused back into the patients (**Figure 5**).

Nevertheless, there are several situations, either *in vivo* or *in vitro*, where cell selection and expansion are not an option, and obtaining a high knockout/gene inactivation efficiency is crucial [26, 27]. Hematological cancer therapies based on specific oncogenic silencing within primitive pluripotent stem cells could be the best example of these situations. In this pathological cell context, the highly efficient interruption of the oncogenic open reading frame (ORF) could be an effective therapeutic option. It would even be more important for those tumors directed by a single oncogenic event, as is the case for several leukemias or sarcomas, which are directed by specific fusion oncoproteins [28, 29].

3. CRISPR-Cas9 technology for disrupting fusion oncogenes

Fusion oncoproteins arising from chromosomal rearrangements are known to drive the pathogenesis of a variety of hematological neoplasms such as CML, which results from a reciprocal translocation between chromosome 9 and 22 [30, 31]. This translocation fuses the *ABL1* gene on chromosome 9 to the *BCR* gene on chromosome 22, resulting in a *BCR/ABL* fusion gene, whose product is a cytoplasmic 210-KDa protein with upregulated tyrosine kinase activity that is considered essential for growth and survival of the leukemic cells [32]. As we previously mentioned, the discovery of *BCR-ABL*-mediated pathogenesis of CML provided the insight for the design of an inhibitory agent that targets BCR/ABL kinase activity such as imatinib mesylate. However, a substantial proportion of CML patients may not achieve the desired response or may eventually fail to respond adequately to these drugs [4]. A recent study of the BCR/ABL oncogen showed this gene fusion to be an ideal target for CRISPR/Cas9-mediated gene therapy. A CRISPR-Cas9 application truncated the specific BCR-ABL fusion (p210) in an *in vitro* cellular model [15] (**Figure 6**).

In this study, a nontumorigenic cell line (BaF3), which needs IL-3 to survive and proliferate [33], was transformed with the fusion oncogene BCR/ABLp210 (BaF3-p210). The human BCR/ABL oncogenic fusion confers on BaF3 the ability to survive and proliferate in the absence of IL-3 and forms tumors in a xenograft model. Three custom-designed sgRNAs were used to genetically inactivate the BCR/ABL oncogene. These specific sgRNAs directed Cas9 to the BCR/ABL fusion sequence (Bcr-Abl sgRNA) or to the Abelson tyrosine kinase sequence (Tk-Abl 1 sgRNA and Tk-Abl 2 sgRNA) (**Figure 7**). Lentiviral infection assays were performed with each CRISPR/Cas9 reagents to generate three different BaF3-p210 cell lines with the potentially edited BCR/ABL oncogene at the expected cleavage point in each one.

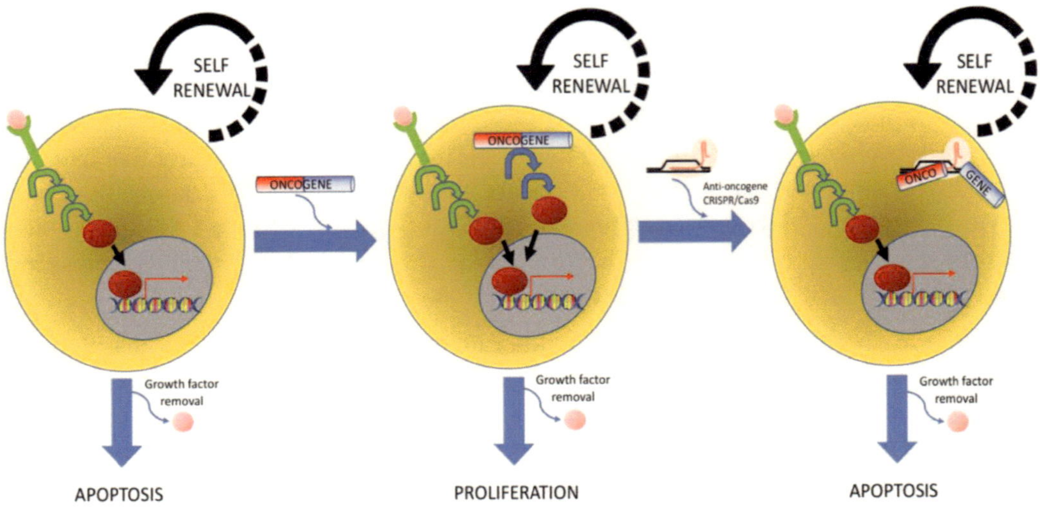

Figure 6. Experimental model to show the ability of CRISPR/Cas9 to truncate BCR/ABL fusion. The non-tumorigenic and IL-3-dependent BaF3 cell line was transformed with fusion oncogene BCR/ABLp210. The transformed cell line is able to grow and survive in the absence of IL-3, although the cells enter into apoptosis when CRISPR/Cas9 introduces mutations in the sequence of the BCR/ABL oncogene, preventing its expression [15].

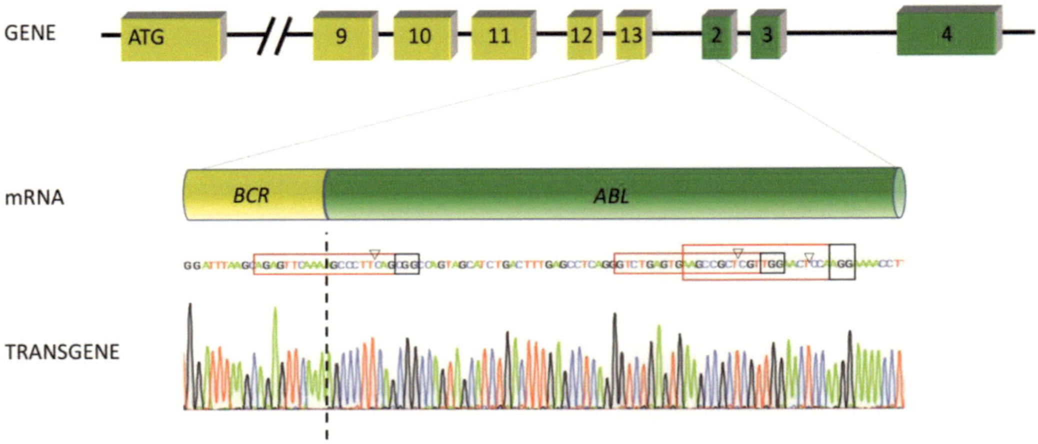

Figure 7. Schematic representation of BCR/ABL fusion transgene. Sequences of sgRNAs designed to edit fusion region (red boxes). One of them hybridizes at the BCR/ABL junction, and the other two hybridize in exon 2 of ABL [15].

The CRISPR/Cas9 system efficiently induced various mutations at the expected cleavage point, giving rise to three distinct BaF3-p210 cell lines (CRISPR-BaF3-p210) with several altered BCR/ABL sequences.

As a result, significantly more cell death was observed in all CRISPR-BaF3-p210 cell lines in the absence of IL-3 than in BaF3 parental cells or mock BaF3-p210 cells (**Figure 8**).

Xenograft experiments were carried out to determine whether the tumorigenic capacity was also blocked by the action of the CRISPR/Cas9 system. Mice injected with the three

http://dx.doi.org/10.5772/intechopen.80245

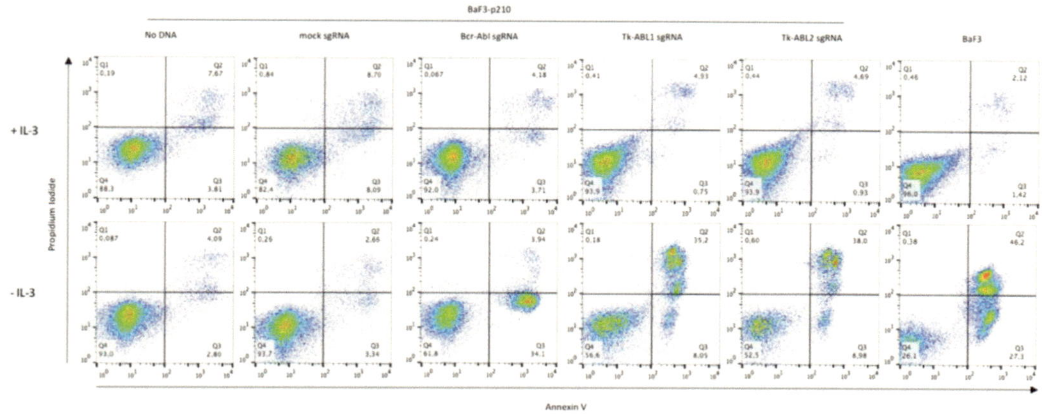

Figure 8. Functional analysis of CRISPR-BaF3-p210-edited cells. Annexin V labeling was measured by flow cytometry in edited cells (BCR-ABL, TK-ABL1 and TK-ABL-2) in the presence and absence of IL-3. When IL-3 was removed from the medium, the three cell lines showed an increase in apoptosis, reflecting the absence of expression of the BCR-ABL oncogene [15].

CRISPR-BaF3-p210 cell lines gave rise to significantly smaller subcutaneous tumors than those produced by the nonedited cells (**Figure 9**).

As expected, these small tumors were composed of nonedited cells, edited cells with +3/−3 bp indels (or multiples), or cells with nonframeshift mutations. This result indicated that a specific cellular selection or more specific sgRNAs should be necessary before potential gene

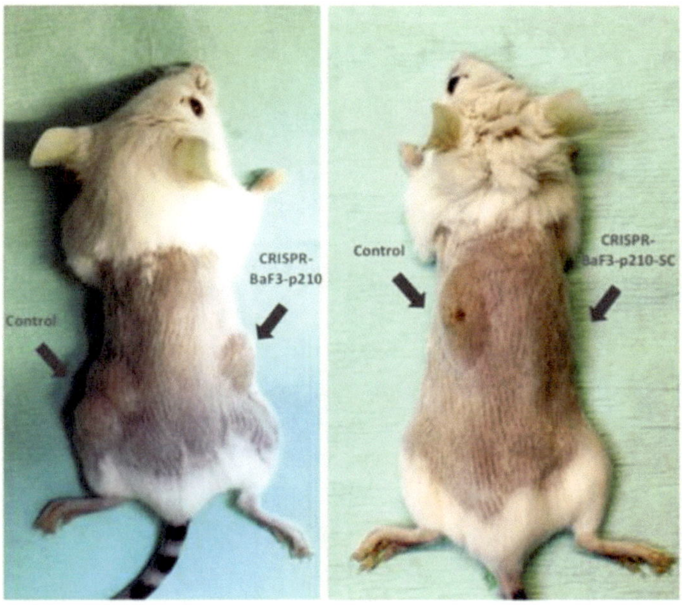

Figure 9. *In vivo* effects of CRISPR-mediated editing of BCR/ABL oncogene. Tumor growth over 24 days following subcutaneous cell injection. The final tumor mass was reduced by half in the CRISPR-BaF3-p210, relative to controls. CRISPR-BaF3 single cell-derived cell line (SC) cells were unable to form a subcutaneous tumor [15].

therapy in human. For this purpose, a CRISPR-BaF3-p210 cell line derived from a single cell (CRISPR-BaF3-p210-SC) carrying an 8-bp deletion (**Figure 9**) was selected to test tumorigenic capacity. No tumor growth was observed in any mouse injected with cells derived from the single-edited cell line (**Figure 9**).

3.1. CRISPR/CAS9 and knocking out genes in mouse

An option to improve knockout effectiveness could be to use two or more RNA guides at the same time to knock out the oncogene allele at different key sites in an attempt to try to guarantee the null result. This approach is commonly used for knocking out genes in animal models such as mice. Using two sgRNA guides makes it possible to distinguish the mutant pups by a simple PCR. An example of this is the generation and genetic characterization of Six6os1-deficient mice [34] (**Figure 10**).

Unfortunately, the possibility of using several RNA guides at the same time is quite limited in gene therapy, especially when adeno-associated virus vectors are used. The main difficulty stems from the limitations on the construct, for which reason other Cas9 orthologues are being used to introduce the nuclease coding sequence, one promoter and a single RNA guide [26, 35].

3.2. CRISPR/Cas9 delivery and gene therapy

The CRISPR/Cas9 complex can be introduced into cultured cells and single-cell embryos in the form of DNA, RNA, or protein [36]. The DNA encoding Cas9 and gRNA can be delivered into the cell using plasmid and viral expression vectors. RNA or protein has been introduced through microinjection, liposome-mediated transfection, electroporation, and nucleofection.

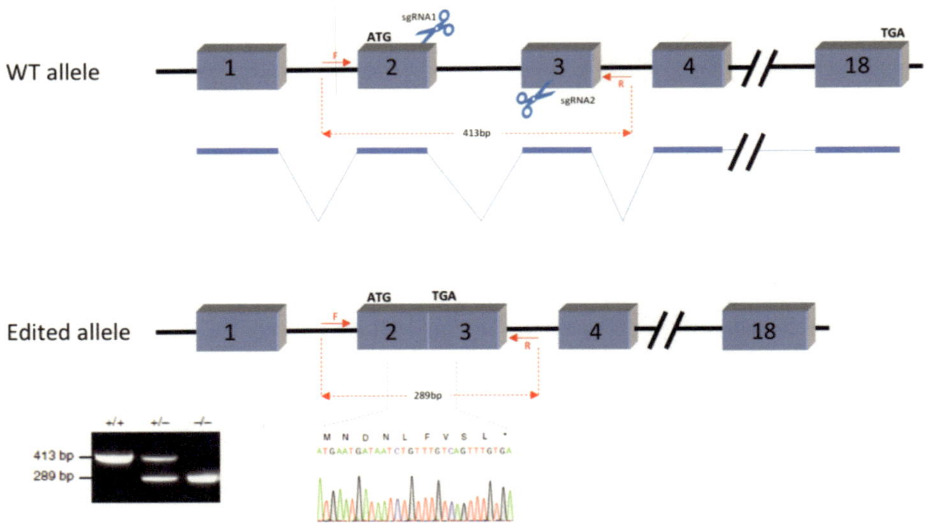

Figure 10. Schematic representation of Six6os1 WT and edited allele. Two sgRNAs were used to produce a deletion between exon 2 and 3. As a consequence, a premature stop codon appears at the beginning of exon 3. The edited allele can easily be detected by PCR [34].

However, the delivery formats of mRNA and protein pose certain technical challenges *in vivo* and viral-based *in vivo* genome editing remain a popular choice for achieving the stable or elevated expression of Cas9 and its sgRNA [37].

Given the great potential of viral vectors in gene and cell therapy, five major classes of viral vectors—retroviruses [38], lentiviruses [39, 40], adenoviruses [41, 42], AAVs [43, 44], and baculoviruses [45, 46]—have been used to deliver CRISPR components into mammalian cells for targeted genome editing. The advantages and disadvantages of using these viral vectors for *in vivo* delivery of the CRISPR transgenes have been extensively reviewed [43, 47–49]. In **Table 2**, we list the general characteristics and applications of various viral delivery vectors.

Currently, adenoviral vectors and γ-retroviruses are the most commonly used delivery system in gene therapy (**Figure 11**; **Table 3**) [1]. For Cas9 delivery, adenovirus (ad)- and retro/lentivirus (rt/lt)-based vectors have the advantage of packaging sizes of up to 30 kb (ad) and 7 kb (rt/lt), allowing the accommodation of the SpCas9 gene (~4.2 kb), one or more sgRNAs, and the cis-acting regulatory sequences required for efficient expression. Nevertheless, several disadvantages such as low titers (rt/lt), insertional oncogenesis (rt/lt), generation of a replication-competent lentivirus (rt/lt), immunogenicity, and toxicity (ad) are risks that should be taken account in *in vivo* gene therapy.

In contrast, the AAV system has major advantages for research and therapeutics, including very low immune response and toxicity. AAVs remain in the cell as episome, avoiding insertional mutagenesis by random integration into the host genome. In fact, there are no human diseases related to them, and they can exist long term as concatemers in nondividing cells for stable transgene expression [50]. Given this, AAV is thought to be one of the most suitable viral vectors for gene therapeutic applications and gene transfer *in vivo*. However, two limitations restrict its use: packing size and tropism. AAV has a packaging capacity of only ~4.8 kb. This makes it impossible to express the ~4.2-kb SpCas9 gene and the sgRNA from a single AAV vector. One approach is to use two AAV vectors: one to express SpCas9 and the other to encode one or more sgRNAs [44]. A second approach is to use a different smaller Cas9, for example, the ~3.2-kb Cas9 gene encoded by *Staphylococcus aureus* (SaCas9) [35, 51]. In this sense, single

Guide	Editing efficiency (%)	TIDE-predicted indels
Bcr-Abl sgRNA	85.0	+1 bp (17.5%), −1 bp (9.1%), −2 bp (4.8%) −3 bp (3.4%), −4 bp (6%), −6 bp (1.8%), −8 bp (18.9%), −11 bp (10.2%), −18 bp (5.1%)
TK-ABL 1 sgRNA	54.6	+1 bp (14.9%), −1 bp (8%) −2 bp (5.2%), −10 bp (17.6%)
TK-ABL 2 sgRNA	68.8	+1 bp (30.8%), −1 bp (5.9%), −2 bp (4.8%), −4 bp (15.2%), −14 bp (5.1%)
Mock sgRNA	0.0	

Table 2. Indels induced by each sgRNA predicted by the TIDE algorithm.

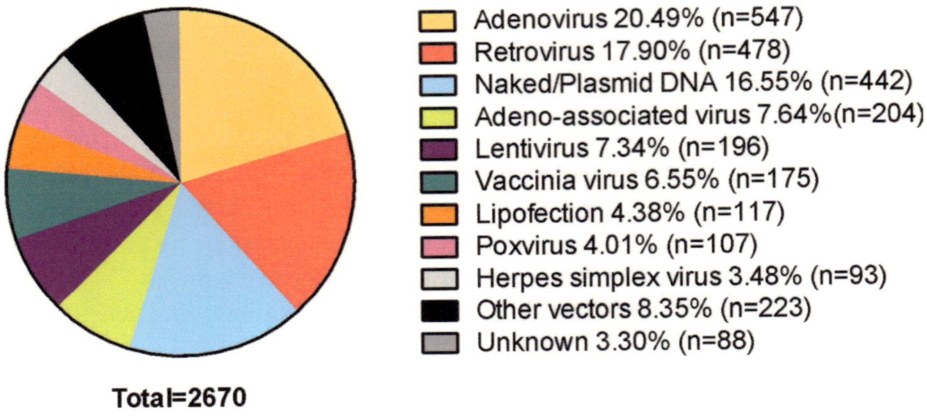

Figure 11. Delivery systems commonly used in gene therapy clinical trials.

Characteristics of a typical vector	Retrovirus	Lentivirus	Adenovirus	Adeno-associated virus	Baculovirus
Common viral type	γ-retroviruses	HIV-1	Ad5	AAV2	AcMNPV
Viral genome structure	Linear ssRNA	Linear ssRNA	Linear dsDNA	Linear ssDNA	Circular dsDNA
Viral genome size	8.3 kb	9.7 kb	36 kb	4.7 kb	80–180 kb
Packaging capacity	<8.0 kb	<8.0 kb	<30 kb	<4.5 kb	>38 kb
Cells infected	Dividing	Dividing or nondividing	Dividing or nondividing	Dividing or nondividing	Dividing or nondividing
Transduction efficiency	Moderate	High	Very high	High	High
Transgene expression	Stable	Stable	Transient	Transient	Transient
Immune response	Moderate	Low	High	Very low	Very low
Toxicity	High	Moderate	High	Low	Low
Random genome integration	Yes	Yes	No	Generally, no (recombinant AAV has a low frequency of host genome integration events)	No
Common applications	Generating stable cell and gene transfer, cancer and stem cell research	Transduce difficult-to-transfect cell, genome-wide screens	Vaccine production, cancer-immune therapy	Gene delivery *in vivo*, optogenetics	Recombinant proteins and vaccine production
Clinical trials	Very popular	Very popular	Popular	Increasingly popular	Growing interest

Table 3. Viral delivery systems most commonly used in gene therapy.

http://dx.doi.org/10.5772/intechopen.80245

AAV vectors are able to express SaCas9, and one sgRNA has been described that appears to be potentially very useful for *in vivo* gene editing. A single AAV vector with U6-driven sgRNA and a TBG-driven SaCas9 expression cassette was used to target the cholesterol regulatory gene Pcsk9 in mouse liver. In this study, the authors observed modification in >40% genes, accompanied by significant reductions in serum Pcsk9 and total cholesterol levels [35].

Another problem with AAV vectors is their limited tissue tropism, although this has gradually expanded with the identification of additional AAV variants from different species and the derivation of AAV recombinants with enhanced tropism for specific tissues [52, 53]. AAV serotypes with a strong tropism for hepatocytes, neurons, and epithelial and endothelial cells have been described, but the search for AAV variants that can efficiently infect HSC or lymphoid cells has yet to identify any candidates [54].

All these advantages have led to increases in the number of studies using AAV vectors to deliver the CRISPR components in animals and in clinical trials for gene therapy.

3.3. CRISPR-Cas9 sgRNAs: "Superguides" for interfering with (onco)gene expression

When a cancer cell is the target, a delivery strategy that can result in the expression of Cas9 and an oncogen-specific sgRNA in all infected cells is desirable. This is especially critical for *in vitro* gene therapy where the expansion processes from a selected edited cell are not available. Similarly, it is also crucial for *in vivo* approaches in cancer therapies focused on disrupting a driver oncogene. If the efficiency of CRISPR/Cas9 reagents delivery to the cancer cell is acceptable, the key step for success lies in the effectiveness of a specific sgRNA at knocking out the oncogene. In this way, for the vast majority of knockout studies where the edited cells or mice can be selected, the sgRNA targets different positions within the chosen exon, avoiding boundaries. In most of these cases, the designs follow off-target criteria. However, for all those cases where cellular selection is not an option and only one sgRNA can be used, the null effect could be increased with a sgRNA targeting the exon boundary. Following this strategy, the generation of null alleles would be increased by two ways: probability of producing a frameshift mutation and probability of breaking the canonical pre-mRNA splicing (**Figure 12**).

It has long been known that mutations in splice-site consensus sequences can affect pre-mRNA splicing patterns and can lead to generate null or deficient alleles [55]. In fact, pioneering genetic studies indicated that many of the thalassemia mutations in the β-globin gene affect splice sites and give rise to aberrant splicing patterns [56, 57]. Recent studies have demonstrated that a splicing mutation in the STAR gene is a loss-of-function mutation that produces an aberrant protein [58]. Besides, non-sense-mediated mRNA decay (NMD), a conserved biological mechanism that degrades transcripts containing premature translation termination codons, could help secure the null effect when a DSB is induced in splice sites. In addition to transcripts derived from nonsense alleles, the substrates of the NMD pathway also include pre-mRNAs that enter the cytoplasm with introns intact [59]. Several mutations of splice donor sites that cause loss of gene function have recently been identified. A novel mutation at a splice donor site that was predicted to lead to skipping of exon 10 of the PLA2G6 gene was found in a homozygous state in infantile neuroaxonal dystrophy patients. This variant was correlated with very strong loss of function, providing further evidence of its pathogenicity [60]. Mutations in the

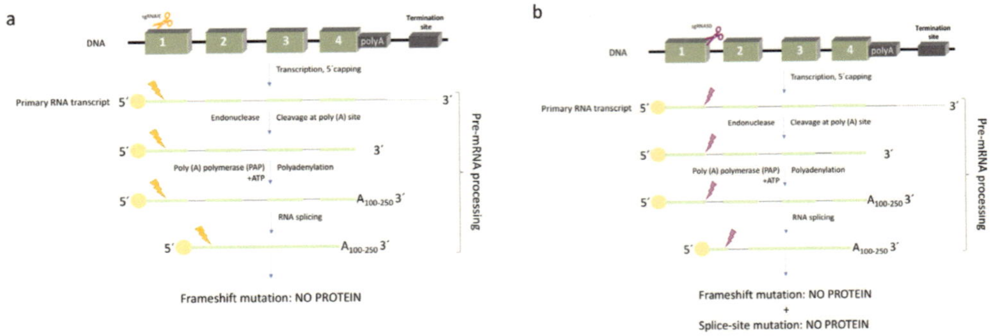

Figure 12. CRISPR/Cas9 design against sequences involved in intron processing.

ectodysplasin A1 gene (EDA-A1) at the splice donor site have been described in patients with hypohidrotic ectodermal dysplasia. The mutation resulted in the production of a truncated EDA-A1 protein caused by the complete omission of exon 3. This novel functional skipping-splicing EDA mutation was considered to be the cause of the pathological phenotype [61]. Studies in a family with premature ovarian failure identified a variant that alters a splice donor site. This variant resulted in a predicted loss of function of the MCM9 gene, which is involved in homologous recombination and repair of double-stranded DNA breaks [62].

As we have mentioned before, not all indels targeting the exon coding sequences necessarily give rise to premature stop codons. However, if DSBs are induced near the boundaries of the target exon, then the canonical splicing pathway could also be altered. In that case, to the probability of producing frameshift, mutations should be added that of interfering with canonical pre-mRNA splicing (**Figure 12B**). Even if the CRISPR/Cas9-induced mutation did not produce a frameshift mutation, at least this strategy would offer the possibility of producing nonfunctional oncogenes by splice-pathway alteration. It has recently been shown that CRISPR/Cas9-mediated alterations at exon boundaries may also result in altered splicing of the respective pre-mRNA, most likely due to mutations of splice-regulatory sequences. Using the human FLOT-1 gene as an example, the authors demonstrated that such altered splicing products also give rise to aberrant protein products with loss of function [63].

An unpublished study has compared the efficiency of generating null alleles by CRISPR/Cas9 sgRNAs targeting exon boundaries. The authors compared the efficiency of producing null alleles inducing DSBs in a central position of the critical exon with DSBs close to the splice donor site on the exon. The study, which was carried out in a variety of genes, species and systems, revealed an increase in knockout efficiency using sgRNA guides targeting the splice-donor site of the chosen exon.

4. Conclusions

Genome-editing nucleases like the popular CRISPR/Cas9 enable knockout cell lines and null zygotes to be generated by inducing site-specific DSBs within a genome. In most cases, when a DNA template is not present, the DSB is repaired by nonhomologous end joining,

http://dx.doi.org/10.5772/intechopen.80245

resulting in small nucleotide insertions or deletions that can be used to construct knock-out alleles. However, for several reasons, these mutations do not produce the desired null result in all cases, giving rise to a similar but functionally active protein. This undesirable effect could limit the therapeutic efficiency of gene therapy strategies that focus on abrogating oncogene expression by CRISPR/Cas9 and should be taken in account. The use of an sgRNA-targeting splicing site could improve the null result for *in vivo* gene therapies. This strategy could be adopted to abrogate *in vivo* the oncogenic activity involved in tumor maintenance.

Acknowledgements

The authors wish to express their sincere thanks to Dionisio Martín, Alberto Pendás (Spanish Research Council, CSIC), for their scientific assistance. We thank all the members at the Transgenic Facility (Nucleus, University of Salamanca), Verónica Alonso and Adrian Montaño for their technical assistance and contribution to our CRISPR/Cas9 studies.

Conflict of interest

The authors declare that they have no conflicts of interest.

Funding

Our CRISPR/Cas9 studies are supported in part by a grant from the Fondo de Investigaciones Sanitarias (FIS) of the Spanish Ministry of Economy (PI17/01895), a Novartis grant, and by the Junta de Castilla y León Fondos FEDER (SA085U16), and to the Programa Propio de Ayuda a la Investigación of the University of Salamanca.

Author details

Ignacio García-Tuñon[1,2], Elena Vuelta[3], Sandra Pérez-Ramos[3], Jesús M Hernández-Rivas[1,2,4], Lucía Méndez[3], María Herrero[3] and Manuel Sanchez-Martin[2,3,4]*

*Address all correspondence to: adolsan@usal.es

1 Centre for Cancer Research (IBMCC), Salamanca, Spain

2 Biomedical Research Institute of Salamanca (IBSAL), Salamanca, Spain

3 Transgenic Facility of Nucleus, University of Salamanca, Salamanca, Spain

4 Department of Medicine, University of Salamanca, Salamanca, Spain

References

[1] Ginn SL, Amaya AK, Alexander IE, Edelstein M, Abedi MR. Gene therapy clinical trials worldwide to 2017: An update. The Journal of Gene Medicine. 2018:e3015

[2] Walther W, Schlag PM. Current status of gene therapy for cancer. Current Opinion in Oncology. 2013;**25**(6):659-664

[3] Sridharan K, Gogtay NJ. Therapeutic nucleic acids: Current clinical status. British Journal of Clinical Pharmacology. 2016;**82**(3):659-672

[4] Ankathil R, Azlan H, Dzarr AA, Baba AA. Pharmacogenetics and the treatment of chronic myeloid leukemia: How relevant clinically? An update. Pharmacogenomics. 2018;**19**(5):475-393

[5] Graham SM, Jorgensen HG, Allan E, Pearson C, Alcorn MJ, Richmond L, et al. Primitive, quiescent, Philadelphia-positive stem cells from patients with chronic myeloid leukemia are insensitive to STI571 in vitro. Blood. 2002;**99**(1):319-325

[6] Duda DG, Kozin SV, Kirkpatrick ND, Xu L, Fukumura D, Jain RK. CXCL12 (SDF1alpha)-CXCR4/CXCR7 pathway inhibition: An emerging sensitizer for anticancer therapies? Clinical Cancer Research. 2011;**17**(8):2074-2080

[7] Nakhlband A, Barar J, Bidmeshkipour A, Heidari HR, Omidi Y. Bioimpacts of anti epidermal growth factor receptor antisense complexed with polyamidoamine dendrimers in human lung epithelial adenocarcinoma cells. Journal of Biomedical Nanotechnology. 2010;**6**(4):360-369

[8] Zhao FJ, Zhang SL, Ma L, Gao H, Zong ZH. Inhibitory effects of c-erbB-2 antisense oligonucleotide transfection on uterine endometrial cancer Ishikawa cell lines. European Journal of Gynaecological Oncology. 2009;**30**(1):54-59

[9] Loriot Y, Mordant P, Brown BD, Bourhis J, Soria JC, Deutsch E. Inhibition of BCL-2 in small cell lung cancer cell lines with oblimersen, an antisense BCL-2 oligodeoxynucleotide (ODN): In vitro and in vivo enhancement of radiation response. Anticancer Research. 2010;**30**(10):3869-3878

[10] Santel A, Aleku M, Roder N, Mopert K, Durieux B, Janke O, et al. Atu027 prevents pulmonary metastasis in experimental and spontaneous mouse metastasis models. Clinical Cancer Research. 2010;**16**(22):5469-5480

[11] Gaj T, Gersbach CA, Barbas CF, 3rd. ZFN, TALEN, and CRISPR/Cas-based methods for genome engineering. Trends in Biotechnology. 2013;**31**(7):397-405

[12] Grimm D, Kay MA. RNAi and gene therapy: A mutual attraction. Hematology American Society of Hematology Education Program. 2007:473-481

[13] Bobbin ML, Rossi JJ. RNA interference (RNAi)-based therapeutics: Delivering on the promise? Annual Review of Pharmacology and Toxicology. 2016;**56**:103-122

[14] Porteus M. Genome editing: A new approach to human therapeutics. Annual Review of Pharmacology and Toxicology. 2016;**56**:163-190

[15] Garcia-Tunon I, Hernandez-Sanchez M, Ordonez JL, Alonso-Perez V, Alamo-Quijada M, Benito R, et al. The CRISPR/Cas9 system efficiently reverts the tumorigenic ability of BCR/ABL in vitro and in a xenograft model of chronic myeloid leukemia. Oncotarget. 2017 Apr 18;**8**(16):26027-26040

[16] Mojica FJM, Montoliu L. On the origin of CRISPR-Cas technology: From prokaryotes to mammals. Trends in Microbiology. 2016;**24**(10):811-820

[17] Jinek M, Chylinski K, Fonfara I, Hauer M, Doudna JA, Charpentier E. A programmable dual-RNA-guided DNA endonuclease in adaptive bacterial immunity. Science. 2012;**337**(6096):816-821

[18] Ceccaldi R, Rondinelli B, D'Andrea AD. Repair pathway choices and consequences at the double-strand break. Trends in Cell Biology. 2016;**26**(1):52-64

[19] Chiruvella KK, Liang Z, Wilson TE. Repair of double-strand breaks by end joining. Cold Spring Harbor perspectives in Biology. 2013;**5**(5):a012757

[20] Karanam K, Kafri R, Loewer A, Lahav G. Quantitative live cell imaging reveals a gradual shift between DNA repair mechanisms and a maximal use of HR in mid S phase. Molecular Cell. 2012;**47**(2):320-329

[21] Heyer WD, Ehmsen KT, Liu J. Regulation of homologous recombination in eukaryotes. Annual Review of Genetics. 2010;**44**:113-139

[22] Simsek D, Jasin M. Alternative end-joining is suppressed by the canonical NHEJ component Xrcc4-ligase IV during chromosomal translocation formation. Nature Structural and Molecular Biology. 2010;**17**(4):410-416

[23] Deriano L, Roth DB. Modernizing the nonhomologous end-joining repertoire: Alternative and classical NHEJ share the stage. Annual Review of Genetics. 2013;**47**:433-455

[24] Wassef M, Luscan A, Battistella A, Le Corre S, Li H, Wallace MR, et al. Versatile and precise gene-targeting strategies for functional studies in mammalian cell lines. Methods. 2017;**121-122**:45-54

[25] Cyranoski D. CRISPR gene-editing tested in a person for the first time. Nature. 2016;**539**(7630):479

[26] Kotterman MA, Schaffer DV. Engineering adeno-associated viruses for clinical gene therapy. Nature Reviews. Genetics. 2014;**15**(7):445-451

[27] Kim E, Koo T, Park SW, Kim D, Kim K, Cho HY, et al. In vivo genome editing with a small Cas9 orthologue derived from *Campylobacter jejuni*. Nature Communications. 2017;**8**:14500

[28] Sanchez-Garcia I. Consequences of chromosomal abnormalities in tumor development. Annual Review of Genetics. 1997;**31**:429-453

[29] Perez-Mancera PA, Sanchez-Garcia I. Understanding mesenchymal cancer: The liposarcoma-associated FUS-DDIT3 fusion gene as a model. Seminars in Cancer Biology. 2005;**15**(3):206-214

[30] Rowley JD. Letter: A new consistent chromosomal abnormality in chronic myelogenous leukaemia identified by quinacrine fluorescence and Giemsa staining. Nature. 1973;**243**(5405):290-293

[31] Rowley JD. Identificaton of a translocation with quinacrine fluorescence in a patient with acute leukemia. Annales de Genetique. 1973;**16**(2):109-112

[32] Ren R. Mechanisms of BCR-ABL in the pathogenesis of chronic myelogenous leukaemia. Nature Reviews Cancer. 2005;**5**(3):172-183

[33] Palacios R, Henson G, Steinmetz M, McKearn JP. Interleukin-3 supports growth of mouse pre-B-cell clones in vitro. Nature. 1984;**309**(5964):126-131

[34] Gomez-H L, Felipe-Medina N, Sanchez-Martin M, Davies OR, Ramos I, Garcia-Tunon I, et al. C14ORF39/SIX6OS1 is a constituent of the synaptonemal complex and is essential for mouse fertility. Nature Communications. 2016;**7**

[35] Ran FA, Cong L, Yan WX, Scott DA, Gootenberg JS, Kriz AJ, et al. In vivo genome editing using *Staphylococcus aureus* Cas9. Nature. 2015;**520**(7546):186-191

[36] Kouranova E, Forbes K, Zhao G, Warren J, Bartels A, Wu Y, et al. CRISPRs for optimal targeting: Delivery of CRISPR components as DNA, RNA, and protein into cultured cells and single-cell embryos. Human Gene Therapy. 2016;**27**(6):464-475

[37] Lau CH, Suh Y. In vivo genome editing in animals using AAV-CRISPR system: Applications to translational research of human disease. F1000Research. 2017;**6**:2153

[38] Williams MR, Fricano-Kugler CJ, Getz SA, Skelton PD, Lee J, Rizzuto CP, et al. A retroviral CRISPR-Cas9 system for cellular autism-associated phenotype discovery in developing neurons. Scientific Reports. 2016;**6**:25611

[39] Koike-Yusa H, Li Y, Tan EP, Velasco-Herrera Mdel C, Yusa K. Genome-wide recessive genetic screening in mammalian cells with a lentiviral CRISPR-guide RNA library. Nature Biotechnology. 2014;**32**(3):267-273

[40] Kabadi AM, Ousterout DG, Hilton IB, Gersbach CA. Multiplex CRISPR/Cas9-based genome engineering from a single lentiviral vector. Nucleic Acids Research. 2014; **42**(19):e147

[41] Wang D, Mou H, Li S, Li Y, Hough S, Tran K, et al. Adenovirus-mediated somatic genome editing of Pten by CRISPR/Cas9 in mouse liver in spite of Cas9-specific immune responses. Human Gene Therapy. 2015;**26**(7):432-442

[42] Cheng R, Peng J, Yan Y, Cao P, Wang J, Qiu C, et al. Efficient gene editing in adult mouse livers via adenoviral delivery of CRISPR/Cas9. FEBS Letters. 2014;**588**(21):3954-3958

[43] Schmidt F, Grimm D. CRISPR genome engineering and viral gene delivery: A case of mutual attraction. Biotechnology Journal. 2015;**10**(2):258-272

[44] Swiech L, Heidenreich M, Banerjee A, Habib N, Li Y, Trombetta J, et al. In vivo interrogation of gene function in the mammalian brain using CRISPR-Cas9. Nature Biotechnology. 2015;**33**(1):102-106

[45] Mansouri M, Ehsaei Z, Taylor V, Berger P. Baculovirus-based genome editing in primary cells. Plasmid. 2017;**90**:5-9

[46] Mansouri M, Bellon-Echeverria I, Rizk A, Ehsaei Z, Cianciolo Cosentino C, Silva CS, et al. Highly efficient baculovirus-mediated multigene delivery in primary cells. Nature Communications. 2016;**7**:11529

[47] Chen X, Goncalves MA. Engineered viruses as genome editing devices. Molecular Therapy. 2016;**24**(3):447-457

[48] Kwang TW, Zeng X, Wang S. Manufacturing of AcMNPV baculovirus vectors to enable gene therapy trials. Molecular Therapy Methods and Clinical Development. 2016;**3**:15050

[49] Epstein BE, Schaffer DV. Combining engineered nucleases with adeno-associated viral vectors for therapeutic gene editing. Advances in Experimental Medicine and Biology. 2017;**1016**:29-42

[50] Kennedy EM, Cullen BR. Gene editing: A new tool for viral disease. Annual Review of Medicine. 2017;**68**:401-411

[51] Friedland AE, Baral R, Singhal P, Loveluck K, Shen S, Sanchez M, et al. Characterization of *Staphylococcus aureus* Cas9: a smaller Cas9 for all-in-one adeno-associated virus delivery and paired nickase applications. Genome Biology. 2015;**16**:257

[52] Kay MA. State-of-the-art gene-based therapies: The road ahead. Nature Reviews. Genetics. 2011;**12**(5):316-328

[53] Zincarelli C, Soltys S, Rengo G, Rabinowitz JE. Analysis of AAV serotypes 1-9 mediated gene expression and tropism in mice after systemic injection. Molecular Therapy. 2008;**16**(6):1073-1080

[54] Smith LJ, Ul-Hasan T, Carvaines SK, Van Vliet K, Yang E, Wong KK Jr, et al. Gene transfer properties and structural modeling of human stem cell-derived AAV. Molecular Therapy. 2014;**22**(9):1625-1634

[55] Krawczak M, Reiss J, Cooper DN. The mutational spectrum of single base-pair substitutions in mRNA splice junctions of human genes: Causes and consequences. Human Genetics. 1992;**90**(1-2):41-54

[56] Treisman R, Orkin SH, Maniatis T. Specific transcription and RNA splicing defects in five cloned beta-thalassaemia genes. Nature. 1983;**302**(5909):591-596

[57] Treisman R, Proudfoot NJ, Shander M, Maniatis T. A single-base change at a splice site in a beta 0-thalassemic gene causes abnormal RNA splicing. Cell. 1982;**29**(3):903-911

[58] Camats N, Pandey AV, Fernandez-Cancio M, Fernandez JM, Ortega AM, Udhane S, et al. STAR splicing mutations cause the severe phenotype of lipoid congenital adrenal hyperplasia: Insights from a novel splice mutation and review of reported cases. Clinical Endocrinology. 2014;**80**(2):191-199

[59] Matsuda D, Sato H, Maquat LE. Chapter 9. Studying nonsense-mediated mRNA decay in mammalian cells. Methods in Enzymology. 2008;**449**:177-201

[60] Elsayed LEO, Mohammed IN, Hamed AAA, Elseed MA, Salih MAM, Yahia A, et al. Case report of a novel homozygous splice site mutation in PLA2G6 gene causing infantile neuroaxonal dystrophy in a Sudanese family. BMC Medical Genetics. 2018;**19**(1):72

[61] Wood-Trageser MA, Gurbuz F, Yatsenko SA, Jeffries EP, Kotan LD, Surti U, et al. MCM9 mutations are associated with ovarian failure, short stature, and chromosomal instability. American Journal of Human Genetics. 2014;**95**(6):754-762

[62] Liu G, Wang X, Qin M, Sun L, Zhu J. A novel splicing mutation of ectodysplasin A gene responsible for hypohidrotic ectodermal dysplasia. Oral Diseases. 2018

[63] Kapahnke M, Banning A, Tikkanen R. Random splicing of several exons caused by a single base change in the target exon of CRISPR/Cas9 mediated gene knockout. Cells. 2016;**5**(4)

Chapter 3

Gene Silencing Agents in Breast Cancer

Amal Qattan

Additional information is available at the end of the chapter

http://dx.doi.org/10.5772/intechopen.79642

Abstract

MicroRNAs (miRs) are a class of non-coding RNAs, approximately 20–25 nucleotides long, discovered in the nematode, *Caenorhabditis elegans*, in 1993. There are two primary categories of non-coding RNA (ncRNA): (1) short interfering RNAs (siRNA) and (2) microRNAs (miRs). In general, miRs control protein production via partially complementary binding of the mRNA 3'UTRs. Both siRNAs and miRNAs are critical regulators of developmental and homeostatic processes as well as disease pathogenesis. While the treatment of advanced stage breast cancer presents several challenges, the development of therapeutic resistance contributes to a high mortality rate. Dysregulation of miR expression has been implicated in progression of breast cancer disease. Moreover, miRs have been found to play a role in the development of drug resistance. In this context, one of the therapeutic potentials of miRNAs is the correlation of circulating miR levels with breast cancer progression stages and disease phenotypes. Secondly, researchers are investigating novel delivery strategies for the substitution or silencing of ncRNAs involved in the disease. This chapter describes both the general miRNA mechanism of actions and the miRNAs related to breast cancer research. It is specifically designed for breast cancer researchers with expertise in gene delivery, clinicians, and clinical translational scientists.

Keywords: microRNA (miRs), short interfering RNAs (siRNA), gene regulation and gene silencing, target recognition, breast cancer, triple negative breast cancer, therapeutic agents, clinical trials, nanoparticle

1. Introduction

Gene silencing by RNA occurs when dsRNA induces cleavage of its complementary mRNA, which is known as RNA interference (RNAi). RNA interference (RNAi) is the mechanism that suppresses gene expression or translation through the activity of RNA interference molecules (RNAi), by the neutralization of mRNA molecules. RNAi is also part of the cell's endogenous biological defense system which protects it against transposons and viruses. miRNAs and siRNAs are vital players in driving RNA interference mechanisms. These small RNAs bind mRNA molecules and either decrease or increase their activity and preventing their translation into protein.

In addition to RNAi, studies have identified several endogenous small RNA types including endogenous siRNA (endo-siRNA), small noncoding RNAs (miRNAs), and piwi-interacting RNA (piRNA) which has created a wider view of normal and pathological cellular mechanisms [1]. The above types are considered non-coding RNAs (ncRNAs) which describes any RNA that does not encode a protein [2, 3]. Since the early 1990s, ncRNAs including miRNAs and siRNAs have been the subject of intensive research. Although non-protein coding RNAs (ncRNAs) were first imagined as simply 'junk' RNA with no functional purpose, they have emerged as potent gene silencing factors [4]. Despite the importance of miRNA in medicine, mechanisms of genes targeting, their interaction with other cellular RNAs, as well as their mRNA editing capabilities are not yet fully understood [5]. It is clear that, the role of ncRNAs in the regulation of genes renders them putative targets for the development of novel drug therapies. As effectors, siRNAs and miRNAs can be used to silence or 'switch off' specific cancer genes. Thus, gene silencing via RNA interference (RNAi) is evolving as an aspect of cancer chemotherapy that could be personalized for individual patients. The therapeutic potential of miRNAs and siRNAs to play a key role in the treatment of cancer and other genetic diseases has been extensively investigated [2]. With the aim of mitigating side effects on healthy tissue, recent approaches have involved the selective targeting of mutant cancer cells.

At present, the main hurdle in implementing miRNA and siRNA therapy in the clinic is the absence of an efficient and targeted delivery system that would protect ncRNAs from degradation by endogenous RNAses and permit them to reach the precise tumor target [6]. Recently, nanoparticle technology and breast cancer targeting immunoconjugates for the delivery of siRNAs and miRNAs were demonstrated to control breast cancer tumor growth and metastasis [7].

MicroRNAs (miRs) are genomically encoded small, non-coding, single stranded RNA 18–25 nucleotides that regulate gene expression during embryonic development. In normal cells they act as a delicate switch in regulating cellular functions such as cell proliferation and cell differentiation [6]. Various preclinical research studies have sought to establish diagnostic, prognostic and therapeutic uses for miRNAs [3]. As a result, downregulated miRNAs in cancer cells are referred to as tumor suppressor miRNAs, while miRNAs that permit the expression of genes involved in cancerous processes are called oncomiRs [1]. siRNAs (with 21–25 nucleotides) are produced from exogenous double stranded (dsRNA); their structure is closely related to that of mature miRNAs. Nevertheless, similarities in the mechanisms and biogenesis of siRNAs and miRNAs have been observed. For example, both depend on Dicer enzymes and on Ago proteins. Most miRNAs, for example, are excised from the precursor (pre-miRNAs) by Dicer while the Ago will support the silencing [8].

2. Molecular mechanisms for triggering silencing through microRNAs

In principle, miRNAs are generated in the nucleus via long primary miRNA transcript (pri-miRs), which are converted by the microprocessor complex into a 70-nucleotide stem-loop structure. This complex consists of Drosha (an RNase III enzyme) and a dsRNA binding protein critical region 8 (DGCR8) DNA sequence. After binding, the dsRNA component of pre-miRNA is cleaved. As partial cleavage occurs, the pre-miRNA is transferred from the nucleus to the cytoplasm through the exportin-5 pathway and further processed by Dicer; the dsRNAs now consists of an inactive passenger strand and an active mature strand. When the 'mature' miRNA is incorporated into the RISC complex it triggers a silencing effect on the target.

With regard to gene silencing and its possible applications in the clinic, miRNA can target multiple sites and thus modulate the expression of many genes. Recognition of mRNA occurs when it binds to a short sequence of nucleotides rather than to the total 21 nucleotides that form an siRNA.

To initiate RNAi, an miR can be partially complementary, binding to multiple mRNAs to block their expression. It is noteworthy that the mechanism of action of an miR is distinct from that of an RNAi in that miRs inhibit the translation of the mRNA [6]. In contrast, a small siRNA is perhaps the most frequently employed RNAi mechanism to silence protein coding genes in the short term. SiRNA is a synthetic RNA duplex structure designed to target specific mRNA in order to degrade it. In the laboratory, gene knockdown is commonly achieved in many cell types using siRNA. Normally, a perfect match is required between the siRNA oligonucleotide and the target mRNA sequence. Finally, siRNA can also be used to knockdown non-protein coding genes e.g. long non-coding RNAs (lnRNA) [9].

siRNAs and miRNAs are highly potent compared to small therapeutic molecules. In addition, both can act on proteins which lack enzymatic functions as well as those which cannot be reached by conventional drug molecules. Currently, two main therapeutic strategies are based on miRNAs, namely: (1) replacement of miRNA or (2) miRNA inhibition. Inhibition of miRNA can be conceptualized as antisense therapy, since synthetic, single stranded RNAs, act as miR antagonists which inhibit the activity of endogenous miRNAs. In contrast, synthetic miRNAs can replicate, substitute, or enhance the function of endogenous miRNAs. Thus, exogenous miR therapy results in mRNA degradation or inhibition leading to gene silencing.

siRNA, for its part involves the introduction of a man-made siRNA into the target cells to trigger RNA interference (RNAi), leading to inhibition of the mRNA expression and thus to gene silencing. Both miRNAs and siRNAs have similar physicochemical characteristics, but their functions are quite separate. Although their mechanisms of action are the same- both are short RNA duplexes that target mRNAs to silence gene, miRNA employs translational repression, the degradation of the mRNA and occasionally, endonucleolytic cleavage of mRNA, while siRNA works exclusively via the endonucleolytic cleavage of target mRNA [2].

3. Challenges in breast cancer diagnosis and treatment

In the Middle East, 25% of all reported cases of female cancer in 2012, were breast cancers. It has been projected that by 2020 about 2 million women will be diagnosed with breast cancer worldwide, a disturb increase of approximately 18.4% [3, 10]. Moreover, about 30% of Middle Eastern patients with newly diagnosed early stage breast cancer will go on to develop metastasis despite extensive therapy [6].

To prevent an advanced stage breast cancer diagnosis, women undergo periodic screening including self-breast examination and yearly mammograms beginning at the age of 40. More frequent monitoring is recommended for women at a high risk of contracting the disease, including those with a family history of it or genetic predisposition [11]. An epidemiological survey concluded in January 2017 reported that female breast cancer is the most frequently diagnosed cancer worldwide [12]. Though the gold standard for detecting breast cancer is mammography, it can cause significant discomfort, and it is not consistently reliable for the detection of smaller tumors at an early stage [3, 13].

3.1. Classification of breast cancer

Breast cancer has been traditionally classified in the clinic as either non-invasive or invasive, according to grade and stage. The classification system is based on the histological features of breast samples as well as the location of abnormal tissues. The two main forms of non-invasive breast cancer are ductal carcinoma *in situ* (DCIS) and lobular carcinoma *in situ* (LCIS). Non-invasive forms remain localized to the breast and do not migrate to nearby tissues and organs. However, most breast cancer are invasive and have been classified as infiltrating ductal carcinoma, tubular carcinoma, invasive lobular carcinoma, medullary carcinoma, inflammatory carcinoma and colloid carcinoma. Breast cancer is considered metastatic if it spreads to the other regions of the body through the blood or lymphatic systems.

Breast cancers are currently classified according to four molecular subtypes: luminal A, luminal B, HER-2 enriched and basal-like cancer. This classification is based on the expression level of the progesterone receptor (PR), estrogen receptor (ER) and the human epidermal growth factor receptor 2 (HER2). Seventy percent of breast cancers are responsive to hormone receptors and present an overexpression (abundance) of either PR or ER receptors or a combination of the two. Luminal A type cancers are known to overexpress the hormonal receptor (ER^{+ve} and/or PR^{+ve} and $HER2^{-ve}$), while luminal B type cancers overexpress all 3 receptors (ER^{+ve}/and/or PR^{+ve} and HER^{+ve}). Luminal A and B cancers are characterized by significant gene expression in the luminal epithelial layers of the mammary glands. However, breast cancers that have been shown to have an abundance exclusively of HER2 are referred to as HER2 enriched and account for about 20% of all cases. Basal-like breast cancers have distinct gene signatures. They are mainly triple negative breast cancer (TNBC), which means that the tumors do not express any hormone receptors. TNBCs are held to account for approximately 10% of all cancers of the breast that are known to have a high mortality rate. mRNA profiling has revealed that to date there are ≥6 identified molecular subtypes of triple negative breast cancer. Variable MiR expression levels are observed in each type. These breast cancer classifications include the immunomodulatory (IM) subtype, luminal androgen receptor (LAR), basal-like (BL1 and BL2), mesenchymal stem cell-like (MSL) and mesenchymal (M) [14].

3.2. Diagnostic approach and treatment of breast cancer

The increasing use of modern adjuvant therapy (systemic) and diagnostic tools has resulted in enhanced treatment of early stage breast cancer patients, producing a substantial increase in the overall survival time from diagnosis. However, improvements in the treatment of relapsed metastatic cancer have been marginal at best. Therefore, there is an urgent demand to develop novel therapies to treat malignant and late stage breast cancer [9, 3]. At present the treatment options include surgery, chemotherapy, immunotherapy, hormonal supplements and radiotherapy [6]. Targeted hormonal therapy is available for patients with breast cancers that have been shown to aberrantly express an excess of receptors for hormones. Studies indicate that hormone receptor type breast cancers have a more favorable prognosis than other types. Hormonal therapies are often prescribed following surgery as an adjuvant treatment. For example, tamoxifen prevents the interaction between hormones and their target receptors, while aromatase inhibitors decrease the levels of circulating hormones. Physicians have administered tamoxifen for more than three decades to treat hormone receptor-positive breast cancer (PR^{+ve}, ER^{+ve} or both). Tamoxifen acts as an estrogen receptor antagonist; it blocks the binding of estrogen with its endogenous receptors. Similarly, herceptin, a human anti-HER2 monoclonal antibody, acts by binding to the HER2 receptor thus preventing the generation of growth factors signals in breast cancer cells. Herceptin and tamoxifen can be given alone or together with chemotherapy drugs such as doxorubicin or paclitaxel and radiotherapy if required. However, the heterogeneity of breast cancers remains a fundamental barrier against the accurate molecular classification of the cancers and the implementation of individualized therapy. It is noteworthy that not all patients with hormone receptor overexpression (ER^{+ve} and/or PR^{+ve}) respond favorably to tamoxifen therapy and not all patients that overexpress HER2 respond to Herceptin indicating the presence of other unknown factors that influence the response to breast cancer treatment.

At present, no effective targeted treatment options are available for triple negative breast cancer (TNBC) patients [6]. The degree of genetic aberrations and the absence of HER2, PR and ER receptors render TNBC patients unresponsive to traditional hormonal therapy. TNBC is all too often resistant to the cancer chemotherapy drugs available at present including paclitaxel and epirubicin, which are platinum-based drugs [2]. The definitions of luminal A and luminal B cancers in the clinic have been set using arbitrary criteria, rather than taking gene expression levels into account. This is probably due to the substantial heterogeneity in ER^{+ve} tumors, which can confound the selection of an appropriate treatment regimen. But the Ki-67 index can distinguish between luminal A and luminal B cancer types. Ki-67 is a protein that is used as a cellular marker for proliferation and may serve to identify a potential fifth molecular subtype, normal-like breast cancer, which is similar to luminal A but is less proliferative, thereby showing decreased Ki-67: (ER^{+ve} /PR^{+ve} /$HER2^{-ve}$ /$Ki67^{-ve}$). Luminal B cancer can also be further subdivided into two subgroups: (ER^{+ve} /PR^{+ve} /$Her2^{-ve}$ /$Ki\text{-}67^{+ve}$) and (ER^{+ve} /PR^{+ve} / $Her2^{+ve}$ /$Ki\text{-}67^{+ve}$).

Nowadays, much research effort has focused on the further sub-classification of breast cancer types, based on gene expression and gene mutations including miRNA signatures. However, the prognostic value of this approach is still not clear [3, 6]. A better understanding of gene expression patterns and genetic mutations should help to determine predictive and prognostic markers and identify novel therapeutic targets that could induce the selective silencing of gene expression [6]. It is known that BRCA1 and BRCA2 genes are mutated in all types of breast cancer including TNBC. The expression of PLK1 has been reported as a possibly important marker for TNBC; in addition TP53, GADPH, HRAS, PCNA, CCND1, BIRC5, MYBL2 and IGFBP6 have been reported as being significantly down-regulated or up-regulated genes that are differentially expressed in TNBC cells compared to normal cells, while other research groups have reported the elevated expression of the AR and EGFR gene among TNBC patients [6].

During the last decade, the targeting of small molecular weight protein kinases and monoclonal antibodies against cell surface receptors has shown great promise in the ongoing struggle against cancer. Unfortunately, many of the key genes that cause cancer are still considered to be 'non-druggable', and as a consequence insufficient research has been applied to targeting them. Most tumors, due to their heterogeneity and their genetic instability are highly unlikely to present a single target that is found suitable for a long term treatment regimen [9]. RNAi has been shown to be able to rapidly and efficiently suppressing the expression of any gene in many cell types, thus highlighting the possibility of treating cancer by drug action on any gene that has been shown to induce cancer.

4. miRNA vs. siRNA for gene silencing in treatment of breast cancer

Current research on the drugs that silence genes has provided important insights into the possible value usefulness of these drugs for the treatment of various types of cancer. A number of mRNA targets, as well as interference in mRNA functions by miRs, will almost certainly make major contributions to our understanding and treatment of many diseases. Thus, the clinical application of miRs as diagnostic biomarkers is developing at a rapid pace, with the gene silencing effect of siRNAs on specific genes making them ideal tools for target identification and validation in drug discovery and development.

4.1. Mechanism of target recognition by miRNA and siRNA

The target recognition of miRNAs is a multifaceted process due to the presence of various binding sites and differing degrees of complementarity between the miRNA and the target mRNA; that is, to induce a functional effect, miRs need to be partially complementary to their target mRNAs. Complementary pairing between mature miRNA and mRNA takes place at the 3'UTR group on the mRNA and the seed region of the miR. In contrast, other miR binding sites, such as the 3′ supplementary sites, centered sites and bulged sites are believed to be aberrant. Therefore, since perfect matching is not required, one miR strand can target an extensive number of mRNAs; thus one miR often has multiple targets. For example, due to partial complementary base pairing between the miR and the mRNA, AGO2, which plays a vital role in RNA silencing, miRISC is not stimulated. Alternatively, the mRNA targets themselves, silence miR via degradation by deadenylation or translation repression via exonucleases or decapping. Rarely, a high degree of complementarity between the miR and its mRNA target may produce endonucleolytic cleavage of the mRNA through the activity of the AGO protein. This activity is quite similar to the gene silencing mediated by siRNA [2]. In contrast, the siRNA must be matched fully with its target mRNA. The activation of AGO2 after complementary binding, leads to the cleavage of the phosphodiester bonds of mRNA bases 10 and 11 relative to the guide strand 5′ end. Any mRNA fragments produced as a result of this activity undergo rapid degradation through the actions of exonucleases [2].

4.2. Role of RNAi technology in breast cancer therapy

In the context of breast cancer therapy, target genes can be silenced by inhibiting miRNA with drugs or by substituting exogenous miRNA. This type of inhibition therapy is deemed useful when tumor cells are known to overexpress the target miRNA. The therapy involves the introduction of single-stranded, synthetic, RNAs that effectively act as miRNA antagonists. In this regard, the inhibition of miRNA is analogous to antisense inhibition. In contrast, cancer be treated by replacing miRNA when the target miRNA is deactivated or repressed, a common feature of cancer. This strategy involves introducing double stranded synthetic miRNAs into cells, which will mimic the actions of the target miRNAs. They bind to the target gene and initiate mRNA degradation which silences the target gene. miRNA mimics are more straightforward to use than siRNA, because the sequences are nearly identical to the endogenous miRNA [6].

In an alternative approach, siRNAs can be produced through gene expression or by chemical synthesis. The strategy governing chemical synthesis is to create synthetic RNAs that can be introduced into cells by a number of methods. The gene expression strategy can produce siRNA using expression constructs, including viral vectors and plasmids, that can be transcribed inside the cell and express short hairpin RNA (shRNAs) that are the precursors of siRNAs. When siRNAs are chemically synthesized this method provides fine control over the purity and quantity of the siRNAs produced. Furthermore, the chemical structure can be modified to improve the stability of the product, which is important when the delivery technique has to be considered. Synthetic siRNAs can also incorporate fluorescence labels using high-resolution fluorescence microscopy to analyze siRNA and its localization in cancer cells [6]. After the introduction of the siRNA into the cell, gene silencing is initiated, a process directed by the endogenous RNAi machinery. Within the cell, duplex siRNAs are incorporated into the RNAi pathway. The antisense strands are loaded onto the RNA induced silencing complex (RISC), which acts as a guide to permit the recognition of complementary mRNAs. Once the target sequence is identified, AGO2 protein, which is a constituent of the

RISC complex, cleaves the mRNA decreasing the protein levels produced by silenced gene. The main advantage of using siRNAs vs. conventional drug therapy is that they exhibit very low toxicity and a high degree of specificity. However, non-specific targets can be affected mainly because the miRNA-like activity of the siRNAs can act at the seed-like sequence of the 5′ end leading to a stimulation of the innate immune system induced by dsRNA [6].

It should be recalled that both siRNAs and mimetics engage with the same related RNAi pathways and interact with the RISC complex. Although siRNA and miRNA appear to be similar in all respects profound differences have been identified. For example, it is known that miRNAs are reproduced as primary miRNA transcripts (pri-miRs) through the activity of miR genes. The controlling nuclear complex partially cleaves the miRNA and resulting stem loop pre-miR is translocated from the nucleus to the cell cytoplasm where it is acted on by Dicer, thus transforming it into dsRNA. The dsRNA now consist of a mature or active strand or may incorporate an inactive "passenger strand". miRNA which is mature then interacts with the RISC complex to silence genes. Short dsRNAs, termed siRNAs, are assemblies of 21- to 23 base pairs, with typically 2 nucleotide overhangs at the 3′ ends, although numerous variations have been detected in their length and the degree of overhang. Structurally, they contain an active guide strand and an inactive passenger strand and can be considered 'exogenous RNAs' that can engage with endogenous RNAi pathways. It should be noted that miRNA often has defective complementarity, usually because of changes in the seed sequence at the 5′ end [6]. This finding stands in stark contrast to siRNA and its target mRNA, where there is a perfect fit (full complementarity) between the two composite molecules.

5. miRNA and its expression in breast cancer

It is well known that in most of the cancer cells studied so far the expression of miRNA has generally decreased. This is not surprising, for miRNAs generally act as tumor suppressors in most cells. Moreover, lower levels of miRNA are found in tumor cells that are poorly differentiated in contrast to those with a higher degree of differentiation. This fundamental finding suggests that global changes in the expression levels of miRNA are intimately associated with the degree of differentiation of aberrant cells. It has been demonstrated recently that a number of miRNAs are expressed at lower levels in tumor-derived cell lines than in the corresponding human tissue. Another study has shown that down-regulation of the expression of miRNA levels in cancer cells resulted in tumorigenesis and that the knockout of Dicer and Drosha, molecules necessary for miRNA biogenesis, led to the complete loss of expression of miRNA. Finally, accelerated growth with enhanced invasive properties occurred when tumor cells were injected into nude mice, strongly suggesting that the loss of miRNA expression leads to enhanced tumorigenesis [7].

Several studies have tackled miRNA profiling and their results indicate that many miRNAs are overexpressed in breast cancer. Although several functions of miRNAs have been investigated, it has become clear that many types of experiment will be required to establish whether miRNAs can be used as novel therapeutic agents or as diagnostic markers. One fact is clear:

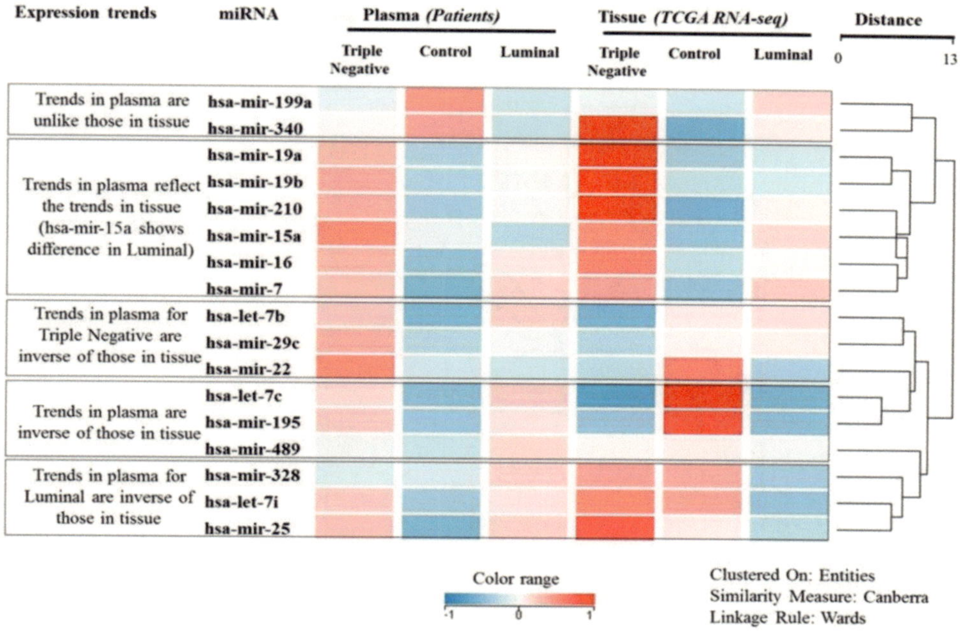

Figure 1. Hierarchical clustering view of the normalized expression levels of miRNA measured in plasma and corresponding miRNA precursor levels in tissue obtained from TCGA RNA-seq data.

tumor metastasis may be promoted through the enhanced expression of pro-oncogenic/pro-metastatic miRNAs or via the down-regulation of anti-oncogenic/anti-metastatic miRNAs. A number of miRNAs have been shown to be deregulated in breast cancer, indicating that particular miRNAs may be involved in the modulation of oncogenesis [3, 15]. miR-10b, miR-125b and miR-145 have been shown to be down-regulated, while miR-21 and miR-155 were up-regulated, strongly suggesting that these miRNAs play important roles as tumor suppressor genes or contribute to creating an oncogene supportive environment [16]. Recently it has been demonstrated that miR-19a, miR-19b, miR-210, miR-15a, miR-16 and miR-7 are overexpressed in plasma as well as in TNBC tissue (**Figure 1**) [3]. At present, a number of research studies have reported on the oncogenic role of miR-19a/b in TNBC tumor development, which occurs due to the repression of PTEN and activation of NF-kB [3, 17]. In addition, the circulating levels of miR-19 have been associated with the efficacy of the epirubicin + paclitaxel chemotherapy regimen in Stage II and III patients with luminal A breast tumors [3, 18]. In a Japanese TNBC patient cohort study, it was reported that a high hsa-miR-210 expression level was an independent risk factor for poor prognosis [3, 19].

6. RNAi as therapeutic in clinical application

In terms of possible clinical applications, a key difference between siRNA and miRNA is that an siRNA specifically targets a single site on a unique mRNA, and initiates inhibition

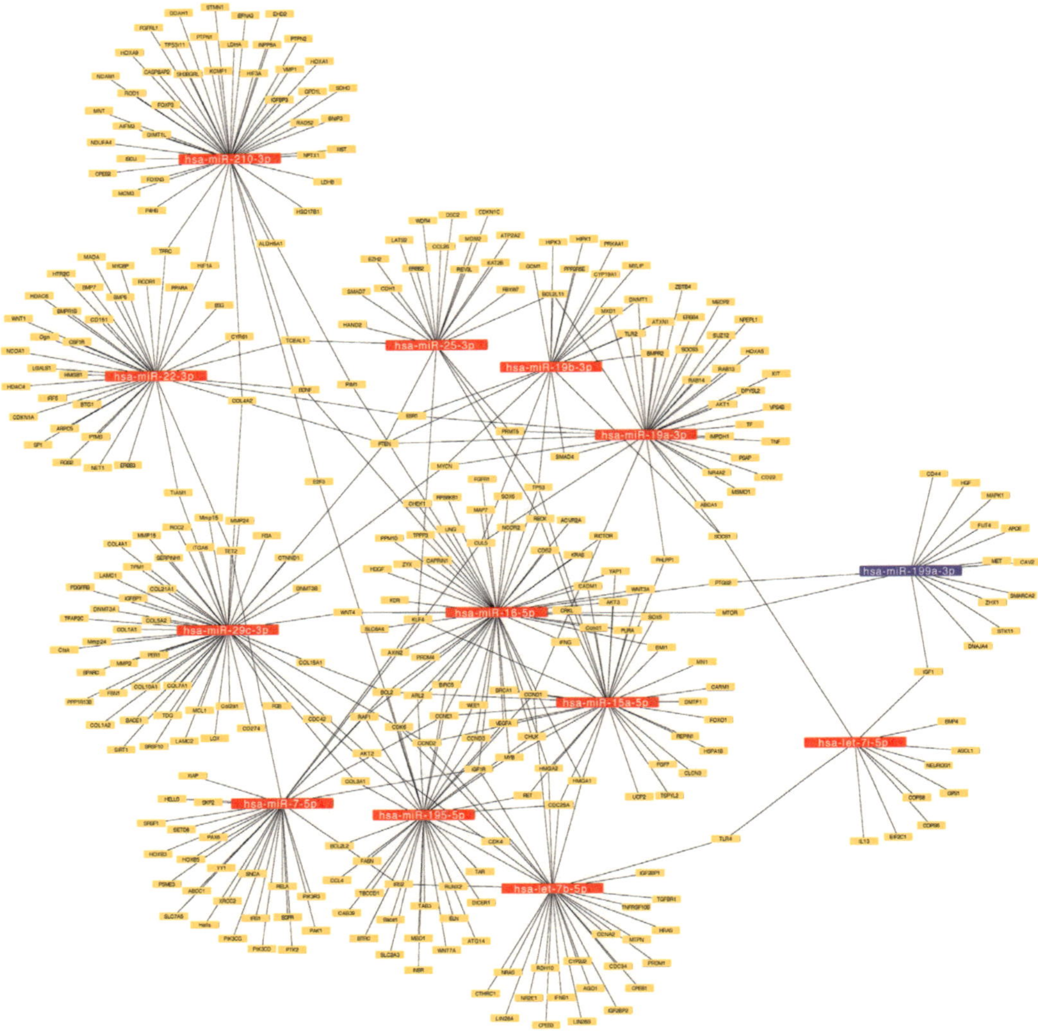

Figure 2. microRNA-mRNA interaction network.

of expression of a single target gene. In contrast, an miRNA molecule usually has multiple mRNA targets and regulates the activity of a number of genes (**Figure 2**). For an mRNA to be recognized by an miR, just a short binding sequence is necessary rather than the entire nucleotide sequence of siRNA. In contrast, the siRNA must be entirely complementary with its target mRNA to enable it to initiate RNAi. However, miRNAs partially complement and bind to multiple mRNAs to inhibit their expression. In addition, their mechanism(s) of action are quite different: siRNAs are known to cleave mRNAs, but miRNAs in contrast act to inhibit the translation of mRNAs. This leads to the inevitable conclusion that scientists will have to develop techniques for targeting specific cells, thus avoiding the down-regulation of the genes expressed by normal cells. The objective will be the delivery of siRNAs and miRNAs to specific targets exclusively in tumor cells. Taken together, three key procedures must be undertaken before RNAi treatment can be given to cancer patients in the clinic, namely: (1) the target gene(s) driving the development of a specific cancer need to be unequivocally identified; (2) an siRNA that specifically targets a particular gene must be fabricated and (3) the man-made siRNA must be capable of being delivered into the target cell cytoplasm [6].

About 20 clinical trials have been initiated to study the great potential of siRNA- and miRNA-based therapy. Only 1 miRNA therapeutic drug, SPC3649, an inhibitor of miR-122, known on the market as miravirsen, has entered clinical trial [20]. A number of other miRNA-based therapeutic agents are currently in the preclinical stage of testing with the aim of introducing the most promising candidates into clinical trials in the near future. At present, many siRNA-based drugs have begun clinical trials for many researchers believe that miRNAs will become a unique category for RNAi-based therapy [20, 21]. The actions of miRNAs are similar to those of siRNAs regarding the post-transcriptional silencing of genes. This chapter has reviewed the biological features of miRNAs and described them as endogenous short RNAs that interact with Argonaute proteins and regulate the expression of many genes. While both siRNA- and miRNA are important for gene regulation at the translational level, endogenous siRNAs help to maintain the stability of the genome. Both are single-stranded and have been shown to be associated with RISC complex components. However, there are fundamental differences between the siRNA and miRNA mechanisms of action. miRNAs most often attach to 8 nucleotides that comprise the 5′ end to enable them to bind to the target mRNA sequences and thus use their inhibitory activity to limit the translation processes. On the other hand, siRNAs use nearly all of their full sequences to identify a particular target and thus mediate cleavage of the targeted mRNA [20]. Taken together, both siRNA and miRNA based therapies are currently under pre-clinical development as breast cancer treatment options.

7. Conclusion

The silencing of gene through RNAi is a natural process that can be found in cells which are mainly involved in the degradation of mRNA and occur in the post-transcriptional phase. Their current status in treatment and diagnosis faces severe challenges because the traditional drugs are not very efficient and also because resistance to the treatment has developed. Silencing the gene that causes this resistance or the genes which cause tumors to form can be regulated by inhibiting them. RNAi i.e., miRNA and siRNA hold great promise in this situation in that these RNAs are involved in silencing the gene. Since their discovery, just over 20 years ago, these genes have been applied as therapeutics and for this they are synthesized synthetically. Not only in cancer, but also in the treatment of other disease as well, they have had a great contributory effect. The genes are very attractive in therapeutic approaches: they have the potential to target any gene in a virtual aspect since they can be synthesized as complementary to their target gene. If compared with conventional drugs, however, their mechanism of action depend on binding with the target site of the target molecule. Though the use of siRNA and miRNA as therapeutics has been found effective, it faces technical barriers such as its delivery to the target tissue, specificity and chemical modification. Delivery to the target tissue requires proper administration to obtain the desired effect. The gene should design carefully, lest it bring about the silencing of other related genes and unwanted effects. A proper safety profile should be maintained in designing the delivery of the RNAi which is highly important for its efficacy. Along with these factors, information regarding silencing effect of the gene, the dosage required for the desired effect, the stability of the RNA molecules, the release of the RNA from the delivery system, and its half-life and turnover of the target proteins are equally important.

Acknowledgements

We would like to thank L'Oréal-UNESCO (FWIS) for their support through a Middle East Fellowship Award (2017) to Dr. Amal Qattan, PhD.

Figure 1 reprinted and adapted with permission from Qattan et al. [3]. Copyright (2017) BMC Cancer Research.

Conflict of interest

The authors declare that they have no competing interest.

Author details

Amal Qattan[1,2]*

*Address all correspondence to: akattan@kfshrc.edu.sa

1 Department of Molecular Oncology, King Faisal Specialist Hospital and Research Centre, Riyadh, Saudi Arabia

2 Department of Biochemistry and Molecular Medicine, School of Medicine and Health Science (SMHS), GW University, Washington, DC, USA

References

[1] Irimie AI, Zimta AA, Ciocan C, Mehterov N, Dudea D, Braicu C, Berindan-Neagoe I. The unforeseen non-coding RNAs in head and neck cancer. Genes. 2018;**9**(3):1-20. DOI: 10.3390/genes9030134

[2] Lam JK, Chow MY, Zhang Y, Leung SW. siRNA versus miRNA as therapeutics for gene silencing. Molecular therapy. Nucleic acids. 2015;**4**:e252. DOI: 10.1038/mtna.2015.23

[3] Qattan A, Intabli H, Alkhayal W, Eltabache C, Tweigieri T, Amer SB. Robust expression of tumor suppressor miRNA's let-7 and miR-195 detected in plasma of Saudi female breast cancer patients. BMC Cancer. 2017;**17**(1):799. DOI: 10.1186/s12885-017-3776-5

[4] Wright MW, Bruford EA. Naming 'junk': Human non-protein coding RNA (ncRNA) gene nomenclature. Human Genomics. 2011;**5**(2):90-98

[5] Li Z, Rana TM. Molecular mechanisms of RNA-triggered gene silencing machineries. Accounts of Chemical Research. 2012;**45**(7):1122-1131. DOI: 10.1021/ar200253u

[6] Ahmadzada T, Reid G, McKenzie DR. Fundamentals of siRNA and miRNA therapeutics and a review of targeted nanoparticle delivery systems in breast cancer. Biophysical Reviews. 2018;**10**(1):69-86. DOI: 10.1007/s12551-017-0392-1

[7] Venugopal ANaSK. Translational research on breast cancer: miRNA, siRNA and immunoconjugates in conjugation with nanotechnology for clinical studies. In: Done S, editor. Breast Cancer – Recent Advances in Biology, Imaging and Therapeutics. InTech Europe: InTech; 2011. pp. 361-380

[8] Carthew RW, Sontheimer EJ. Origins and mechanisms of miRNAs and siRNAs. Cell. 2009;**136**(4):642-655. DOI: 10.1016/j.cell.2009.01.035

[9] Shen H, Mittal V, Ferrari M, Chang J. Delivery of gene silencing agents for breast cancer therapy. Breast Cancer Research. 2013;**15**(3):205. DOI: 10.1186/bcr3413

[10] Albeshan SM, Mackey MG, Hossain SZ, Alfuraih AA, Brennan PC. Breast cancer epidemiology in gulf cooperation council countries: A regional and international comparison. Clinical Breast Cancer. Jun 2018;**18**(3):e381-e392. DOI: 10.1016/j.clbc.2017.07.006

[11] Coughlin SS, Ekwueme DU. Breast cancer as a global health concern. Cancer Epidemiology. 2009;**33**(5):315-318. DOI: 10.1016/j.canep.2009.10.003

[12] Siegel RL, Miller KD, Jemal A. Cancer statistics, 2017. CA: A Cancer Journal for Clinicians. 2017;**67**(1):7-30. DOI: 10.3322/caac.21387

[13] Weinberger M, Saunders AF, Samsa GP, Bearon LB, Gold DT, Brown JT, Booher P, Loehrer PJ. Breast cancer screening in older women: Practices and barriers reported by primary care physicians. Journal of the American Geriatrics Society. 1991;**39**(1):22-29

[14] Qattan A. Metabolic reprogramming of triple-negative breast cancer: The role of miRNAs. MicroRNA Diagnostics and Therapeutics. 2017;**3**:1-8. DOI: 10.1515/micrnat-2017-0001

[15] Lu J, Getz G, Miska EA, Alvarez-Saavedra E, Lamb J, Peck D, Sweet-Cordero A, Ebert BL, Mak RH, Ferrando AA, Downing JR, Jacks T, Horvitz HR, Golub TR. MicroRNA expression profiles classify human cancers. Nature. 2005;**435**(7043):834-838. DOI: 10.1038/nature03702

[16] Iorio MV, Ferracin M, Liu CG, Veronese A, Spizzo R, Sabbioni S, Magri E, Pedriali M, Fabbri M, Campiglio M, Menard S, Palazzo JP, Rosenberg A, Musiani P, Volinia S, Nenci I, Calin GA, Querzoli P, Negrini M, Croce CM. MicroRNA gene expression deregulation in human breast cancer. Cancer Research. 2005;**65**(16):7065-7070. DOI: 10.1158/0008-5472.CAN-05-1783

[17] Mathe A, Scott RJ, Avery-Kiejda KA. miRNAs and other epigenetic changes as biomarkers in triple negative breast cancer. International Journal of Molecular Sciences. 2015;**16**(12):28347-28376. DOI: 10.3390/ijms161226090

[18] Li Q, Liu M, Ma F, Luo Y, Cai R, Wang L, Xu N, Xu B. Circulating miR-19a and miR-205 in serum may predict the sensitivity of luminal A subtype of breast cancer patients to neoadjuvant chemotherapy with epirubicin plus paclitaxel. PLoS One. 2014;**9**(8):e104870. DOI: 10.1371/journal.pone.0104870

[19] Toyama T, Kondo N, Endo Y, Sugiura H, Yoshimoto N, Iwasa M, Takahashi S, Fujii Y, Yamashita H. High expression of microRNA-210 is an independent factor indicating a poor prognosis in Japanese triple-negative breast cancer patients. Japanese Journal of Clinical Oncology. 2012;**42**(4):256-263. DOI: 10.1093/jjco/hys001

[20] Chakraborty C, Sharma AR, Sharma G, Doss CGP, Lee SS. Therapeutic miRNA and siRNA: Moving from bench to clinic as next generation medicine. Molecular Therapy. Nucleic Acids. 2017;**8**:132-143. DOI: 10.1016/j.omtn.2017.06.005

[21] Hydbring P, Badalian-Very G. Clinical applications of microRNAs. F1000Research. 2013;**2**:136. DOI: 10.12688/f1000research.2-136.v3

Chapter 4

Nontransformative Strategies for RNAi in Crop Protection

Deise Cagliari, Ericmar Avila dos Santos,
Naymã Dias, Guy Smagghe and Moises Zotti

Additional information is available at the end of the chapter

http://dx.doi.org/10.5772/intechopen.80874

Abstract

RNAi in crop protection can be achieved not only by plant-incorporated protectants through plant transformation (transgenic) but also by nontransformative strategies such as formulations of sprayable dsRNAs used as direct control agents, resistance factor repressors, or developmental disruptors. Therefore, the RNAi-based biopesticides are expected to reach the market also in the form of nontransgenic strategies such as sprayable products, stem injection, root drenching, seed treatment, or powder/granule. While the delivery of dsRNA by transgenic expression is well established, it requires generations of crop plants and is costly, which may take years and delays for practical application, depending on the regulatory rules, plant transformability, genetic stability, and public acceptance of genetically modified crop species. DsRNA delivery as a nontransgenic approach was already published as a proof-of-concept work, so it is time to point out some directions on how the real potential for agriculture and crop protection is.

Keywords: RNAi-based, biopesticides, nontransgenic approaches, dsRNA, nontransformative plant protection

1. Crop protection and RNAi

The beginning of human civilization can be traced back to the ability of cultivating crops. This has allowed that a higher number of people could be supported in the same environment; however, it also brought several crop protection challenges that mankind has been facing continuously. To ensure sufficient food production, since the earliest days of agriculture, farmers have had a history of using agrochemicals to protect their crops against yield loss from a vast range of organisms including pest insects, mites, fungi, weeds, and others.

The modern era of synthetic pesticides began in the 1930s, and with insects, fungal pathogens, and weeds, destroying each one more than 13% before harvest and about 10% in postharvest [1], the pesticide use has become fundamental to modern crop protection technology. The increasing resistance [2] of weeds, pest insects, and fungi to established agrochemical compound classes, stringent regulatory environment rules, and market growth has stimulated demand for more selective, safer, and cost-effective pest control methods. Crop protection scientists have allocated a great deal of intellectual energy into seeking of more refined strategies to reduce crop losses such as transgenic crops expressing *Bacillus thuringiensis* (Bt) [3] toxins and more recently gene silencing through RNAi (RNA interference) [4, 5].

RNAi is a natural process present in eukaryotic cells for gene regulation and antiviral defense. Although, from a crop protection perspective, RNAi refers to double-stranded RNA (dsRNA)-mediated gene silencing that involves the blocking of the expression of specific target genes by destroying the corresponding mRNA molecules affecting only the translation process. Due to its sequence-dependent mode of action, the RNAi technology, as referred nowadays by industry, has a vast range of potential crop protection application, including genetic studies and pest control research in insects [6–12], mites [13–15] and ticks [16], plant pathogens [17–23], termites, nematodes, and weeds [2, 24, 25] in a range of crops. These RNAi practical applications have been pursuing over the last decade for the development of novel crop protection methods.

The application of this technology did not go unnoticed in agriculture; hence, since the discovery of RNAi and its regulatory potentials, it has become evident that RNAi has immense potential in opening a new vista for crop protection. Nevertheless, one of the biggest challenges for the RNAi technology is to make possible that target organisms (i.e., pest insects, plant pathogens, nematodes, viruses) uptake intact and active molecules that will trigger an RNAi pathway. Delivery of dsRNA to a target organism is the easiest through transformative RNAi approach (i.e., transgenic plants) [26, 27], but it is not practical to every target and crop. Therefore, the development of nontransformative approach (i.e., sprayable dsRNA) [9, 11, 28] for RNAi delivery will boost up its use in the field.

2. RNAi mechanism in brief

The cellular mechanics of gene silencing by RNAi was largely misunderstood or even unknown until the work of Andrew Fire and Craig Mello with the nematode *Caenorhabditis elegans* [5]. RNAi regulates gene expression through small noncoding RNAs (sRNAs). The sRNAs of ~21–25 bp long dsRNA molecules have ~2 nt 3′ overhangs that allow them to be recognized by enzymes from the RNAi machinery, which subsequently leads to homology-dependent degradation of target mRNA. There are two primary classes for sRNAs in the RNAi pathway, the micro-RNAs (miRNAs) and the short-interfering RNAs (siRNAs). The miRNAs are derived from endogenously expressed products and from stem-loop precursors with incomplete double-stranded character, whereas siRNAs are primarily exogenous in origin from viruses or transposons and from long, fully complementary double-stranded RNAs (dsRNAs) [29]. Briefly, both siRNA and miRNA molecules are initially generated from longer dsRNAs processed by the ribonuclease III enzyme dicer into 20–30 nucleotide duplexes. Subsequently, an argonaute family protein (AGO), which is the catalytic component of the RNA-induced silencing complex (RISC), is incorporated. The RISC mediates either the degradation of mRNA or the repression of translation. In most RNAi-competent eukaryotes, with notable exceptions of insects and vertebrates, the primary dsRNA trigger induces the synthesis of secondary siRNAs through the action of RNA-dependent RNA polymerase (RdRP) enzymes. The three classes of molecules, namely dicer, argonaute, and 20–30 nucleotide duplexes of RNA, are heralded as the signature components of RNA silencing of genes, comprehensively reviewed in several articles [8, 9, 12, 29–35].

3. Transformative versus nontransformative RNAi

As aforementioned for field applications, the transformative RNAi includes the plant-incorporated protectants (PIPs; i.e., transgenic plants/RNAi-based plant traits), whereas non-PIP dsRNA-containing end-use products (dsRNA-EPs) might be formulated as dsRNA active ingredient such as a raw material for insecticide, antifungal, or antiviral with variable delivery modes (see Section 4).

The RNAi mechanism works at mRNA level exploring a sequence-dependent mode of action, which makes it unique in potency and selectivity compared to any regular agrochemicals. Therefore, one advantage of RNAi either by transformative or by nontransformative approach is that it would allow farmers to target pests more specifically. The technology can be designed by using sequences of RNA that match very specific gene sequences in a target pest; hence, RNAi should leave other species unharmed. The careful selection of unique regions of pest genes results in effects highly targeted, avoiding unintended effects.

The transformative RNAi strategy through transgenic plants known as host-induced gene silencing (HIGS) has proved to be successful in the protection of crops against their specific pest insects [26, 36–38], plant pathogens [18, 19], viruses [22, 39–41], and nematodes [42, 43], recently reviewed [44].

A proof-of-concept milestone paper of Baum et al. [36] demonstrated that a dsRNA construct in a genetically engineered plant could provoke larval mortality in western corn rootworm (WCR), *Diabrotica virgifera*. This research was fundamental to spread the idea on the potential of dsRNA as a new pest control agent through transgenic plants. In September 2016, the Canadian Food Inspection Agency (CFIA) had announced the approval of the RNAi-based corn event Monsanto MON87411, the "SmartStax PRO" (expressing Cry3Bb1, Cry34Ab1/Cry35Ab1, and DvSnf7) [38], containing a *D. virgifera* dsSnf7 construct in combination with two *Bt* constructs, for commercialization and release. Also, the US EPA had confirmed in June 2017 the approval of this event for commercial planting.

The development of a transgenic plant expressing dsRNA as a strategy for plant protection is straightforward, but it is not practical to every pest organism and crop [9, 10, 12]. Although the delivery of dsRNA by transgenic expression is well established, it requires generations of crop plants, which may take years and delays for practical application, depending on the regulatory rules, plant transformability, genetic stability, and public acceptance of genetically modified (GM) crop species [45].

While RNAi-based crops are expensive to produce and have a high risk of resistance breakdown, topical application is underway as a nontransformative approach that might enable RNAi-based pest management. Therefore, triggering an RNAi pathway in a pest organism may also be possible through a spray-induced gene silencing (SIGS) approach, without changing the plant DNA. The SIGS as a nontransgenic approach for pest control was already published [46] as a proof-of-concept work and recently reviewed [9, 11]. Because of using this approach to silence genes without introducing heritable changes into the genome, it may not be regulated as a GM product. A dsRNA spray can be used almost immediately as a regular pesticide without having to go through several years involved in the development of a GM or conventionally bread crop. Besides, in several countries due to the slow regulatory procedure to approve transgenic crops, nontransformative RNAi strategies with similar results such as some of those demonstrated above could be applied. Still, the main drawback of nontransformative RNAi strategy is that as a plant grows, new leaves have to be sprayed to guarantee protection, so this implies in possible higher costs to farmers, whereas transgenic plants will produce dsRNA continuously. However, the vascular system of plants naturally translocates RNAs [47]. Therefore, sprays on leaves, injection in trunks, or soil application of dsRNA can travel long distances through plant vessels; hence, this can be exploited for the development of pest control strategies [11, 28].

The idea to use sprayable dsRNA was followed by an underlying supposition that this type of molecule would have a short half-life for an effective crop protection agent [48], and the short half-life of dsRNA in soil and by UV light has been confirmed [10]. This apparent challenge posed by SIGS approach is that the effects on plants last only a few days because unprotected RNAs break down soon. Farmers may not want to apply extensive sprays to keep plants protected; however, there are some positive issues because the sprays of dsRNA can be quickly tailored toward a pest organism, much faster than a GM crop, and last only a few days or weeks different from most regular pesticides. Crop protectors should bear in mind that there is no need for a pest control agent persist active for months to become an efficient pest control agent.

Regardless of the target species, for a successful nontransformative RNAi strategy, it is of paramount importance to identify unique regions in very essential target genes, so that brief changes in the level of expression can provoke severe consequences as well as delivery of sufficient amount of intact dsRNA. Alternatively to transgenic plants, the delivery of dsRNA can be through other routes including dsRNA sprays, dsRNA expression in bacteria, trunk injection, and engineered viruses, among others. For example, to control plant viruses, farmers are obligated to either grow varieties with resistance to viruses or try to kill the organism that spread, such as aphids or hemipterans. Sprays with dsRNA might be rapidly tailored against existing or new type of virus, and the gene-silencing effects of RNAi will last only a few days, enough to suppress virus replication. Overall, the SIGS approach opens up a range of possibilities for several pest insects that are difficult to control such as root-feeding and sap-feeding

http://dx.doi.org/10.5772/intechopen.80874

insects, plant viruses, and plant pathogens, especially in perennial crops (e.g., fruits such as grapes, apples, and citrus), where plant transformation takes years to develop and is costly.

4. Successes of RNAi through nontransformative approaches

The delivery of dsRNA through nontransformative approaches is likely to hit the market in four categories: (i) direct control agents; (ii) resistance factor repressors; (iii) developmental disruptors; and (iv) growth enhancers [9–11, 49–52]. As a direct control agent, nontransgenic approaches were successfully managed to achieve long-lasting gene silencing [9, 10, 18, 19, 41].

In some experiments, full-sized citrus and grapevine trees were treated with dsRNA using foliar sprays, root drenching, or trunk injections. Two hemipteran insects, a xylem- and a phloem-feeding, and a coleopteran chewing insect took up the dsRNA after feeding on plants previously treated with dsRNA [11, 28]. Similarly, rice plants were able to take up dsRNAs when their roots were soaked in dsRNA solution showing resistance against piercing-sucking and stem-borer pest insects [53] and also mites [15]. Altogether, these experiments are clear demonstrations that drench/soak roots, trunk injections, and sprays on leaves are success strategies for delivery of dsRNA molecules without any modification on plants DNA.

Plant diseases caused by virus have a tremendous impact in food production and quality, being responsible for loses in several crops, fruits, and vegetables worldwide. Coherent with an ancient role to protect genome from invasive viruses, the RNAi mechanism can be reprogrammed to work by destroying any virus RNA. Without viral RNA, no viral proteins are made, thus preventing virus replication and plant diseases. Some studies have already been conducted on topical application of dsRNA to control plant viruses [41, 54]. However, a major limitation in the practical application of dsRNA to control viruses is that RNAs face a hostile environment where it is rapidly degraded with not only low uptake into plants, but also the short virus protection window of few days postspray. There are some rumors that the initiated pipeline branded "BioDirect" by Monsanto controls pest insects and plant viruses with sprays of dsRNA, but details on this probably are not publically available. To address some of these limitations, a layered double hydroxide (LDH) clay nanosheet, called "BioClay," was developed [55] and combined with dsRNA molecules. The clay nanoparticles are positively charged and so bind and protect the negatively charged RNAs; delivery occurs when atmospheric carbon dioxide and moisture react with clay nanoparticles breaking down LDH, gradually releasing RNAs. Using this dsRNA-LDH complex was possible to achieve long-lasting gene silencing, protecting tobacco plants from a virus for 20 days with a single spray [55, 56], thus extending the period of 5–7 days using naked dsRNA. The complex dsRNA-LDH protected plants in both local lesions and systematically. Also using RNAi to control plant viruses, the mechanism of dsRNA uptake into the leaf was investigated. It was reported a rapid systemic spread of dsRNA when leaves of *Nicotiana tabacum* cv. Xanthi were mechanically inoculated with naked dsRNA homologous to tobacco mosaic virus (TMV) [57]. From these experiments, we can conclude that topical application of dsRNA targeting virus genes can induce a systemic RNAi toward virus resistance.

Direct spray of dsRNA was also used experimentally to control the Colorado potato beetle (CPB), *Leptinotarsa decemlineata,* under greenhouse conditions [10]. The naked dsRNA molecules in foliar application were sufficiently stable for at least 28 days, enough to control the CPB. The authors also investigated the RNA degradation under UV light, where they concluded that an exposition of 1–2 h is needed for dsRNAs to become inactive in feeding assays. The long biological activity (28 days) during greenhouse feeding experiments suggests that naked dsRNA is more stable in leaf surface than in a glass surface used for the UV stability studies.

The fungi kingdom consists of a large and diverse group of eukaryotes, and plant diseases caused by fungi exert particular and agronomic impact on global grain and food production. Generally, the proteins dicer, argonaute, and RdRP, which are some of the major components of RNAi pathways, are present in most fungi species [58]. Therefore, the RNAi pathways can be harnessed to control plant diseases [22]. Sprays of CYP3-dsRNAs, targeting simultaneously three fungal ergosterol biosynthesis genes (P450 lanosterol C-14α-demethylases—*CYP51A, CYP51B, CYP51C*), on barley leaves were used to control *Fusarium graminearum* infections in the local areas, where dsRNA was sprayed, but strikingly also in unsprayed distal leaf parts, showing that dsRNA was systematically translocated within the plant [18]. The example above was a proof-of-concept article showing that after spray an even long dsRNA molecule (791 nt) could be taken up by the plant and transferred as unprocessed dsRNA via plant vascular system to infection sites, where it was processed by the fungal RNAi machinery to carry out its antifungal activity. The same authors also demonstrated that green fluorescent protein (GFP) from jellyfish was silenced in a *Fusarium graminearum* strain expressing GFP, suggesting that sprays of dsRNA are not sequence selective and thus with the potential for targeting any gene across several plant pathogens. Similar study [19] showed that dsRNA and sRNAs targeting dicer-like protein genes DCL1 and DCL2 of *Botrytis cinerea* were externally applied on fruits, vegetables, flower petals, and *Arabidopsis* leaves, followed with *B. cinerea* infection. The authors showed that *B. cinerea* was able to take up dsRNA and sRNAs from the environment, inhibiting gray mold disease.

The study with full-sized citrus trees (2.5 m tall) was performed with 2 g of dsRNA in 15 l of water applied by root drench and injections [46]. The dsRNA was detected in psyllids and leafhoppers 5–8 days postingestion from plants and for at least for 57 days in the citrus trees; this allows the development of an area-wide pest suppression approach. Similarly, Koch et al. [18] showed that the CYP3-dsRNA labeled with the green fluorescent dye (ATTO 488) was detected in the vascular tissue 24 h after spraying leaves. Also, the leaf sections demonstrated that the fluorescence was detected in the xylem, in the apoplast and symplast of phloem parenchyma cells, companion cells, mesophyll cells, as well as in trichomes and stomata. The labeled dsRNA was detected also inside fungal conidia and germ tubes as well as in the fungal mycelium. These experiments conducted by Koch et al. [18] using sprays on barley leaf surface are the first examples of active dsRNA uptake by plant cells.

The uptake of RNAs from the environment, a phenomenon known as environmental RNAi [8], has not yet been observed in mammals. This phenomenon was observed in *C. elegans*, others nematodes and insects [10, 59]. However, until recently, it was not clear whether plants and fungi could take up RNAs from the environment. From what we know so far, it is worth noting that plants and fungi are indeed capable to take up dsRNAs and sRNAs applied externally [18, 19]. As described above, the locally applied dsRNA can inhibit pathogen growth also at distal unsprayed leaves, so these RNAs should be able to spread systematically across plant cells and tissues [18, 55, 60]. The nematode *C. elegans* is able to take up environmental dsRNAs that are longer than 50 bp, where the shorter dsRNAs cannot be taken up [59]. Generally, plant-feeding insects are able to take up dsRNAs that are longer than 50–60 pb, but not shorter dsRNAs or sRNAs [61, 62], while fungi and plants can take up both external sRNAs and long dsRNAs [18, 19]. The differences in the uptake of RNA species between plants/fungi and insects suggest that entry/uptake channels or pathways may differ among organisms. In the light of this, the uptake mechanisms that the externally applied RNAs may be translocated into plant pathogens and/or herbivorous insects could have at least two possible routes for entry. First, for insects, RNAs could be directly taken up during herbivory or through the cuticle to get into insect cells; similarly for fungi, RNAs could be taken up directly into fungal cells after spray. Second, the RNAs could be taken up by plant cells first and then move into insect/fungal cells indirectly (**Figure 1**).

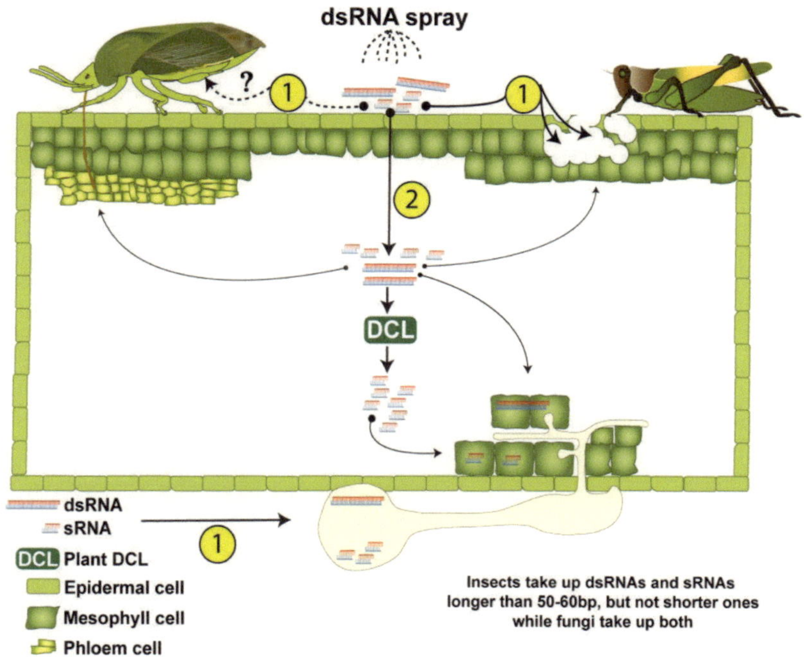

Figure 1. Two possible pathways of silencing insect and fungal genes induced by sprays of dsRNAs and sRNAs. There are at least two possible routes for RNAs to get into insect/fungal cells. Pathway 1: Insects and fungi directly take up sprayed RNAs. The up taken dsRNAs may be sliced into sRNAs by fungal or insect DCL proteins. Pathway 2: Externally applied dsRNAs and sRNAs are taken up by plant cells and then transferred into insect or fungal cells. The long dsRNAs may be sliced into sRNAs by plant dicer like (DCL). In both possible pathways, fungi take up longer and shorter dsRNAs, while insects take up dsRNAs longer than 50–60 bp in length. For phloem-feeding insects such as stinkbugs and aphids, sprayed RNAs may prove difficult to get into insect cell directly (pathway 1), while for chewing insects such as grasshoppers and caterpillar, RNAs are taken up easily during herbivory.

One obstacle, if not the biggest, is the cost for the mass production of dsRNA. While the issues of environmental stability and delivery are being addressed with creative innovations such as BioClay, making mass amounts of RNA is still expansive. Indeed, cost-effective methods will allow real-world applications of exogenous dsRNA for RNAi-mediated crop protection. To our knowledge, currently, there are no commercial RNAi-based products that utilize dsRNA as a spray for crop protection. Since the discovery of dsRNA and its potential for crop protection, some companies and academic scientists are seeking to develop more cost-efficient methods for large production of dsRNA. Similarly, RNAi to control devastating pests such as the Colorado potato beetle has obviously attracted attention in private research and development. As mentioned before, Monsanto (currently Bayer) and Syngenta (current ChemChina) have allocated major investments toward SIGS technology. Already in mid-2015, Monsanto launched its technology BioDirect, and although the principle was the same as we had seen in academia, these products work differently because they are not expressed in the leaves, but applied exogenously to the plants. Syngenta scientists also are developing lines of biocontrol products based on RNAi (https://www.youtube.com/embed/BiVZbAy4NHw?ecver=1). For example, these dsRNA-based products when sprayed onto the potato plants (field trials) or soy plants targeting genes of Colorado potato beetle and stink bug, *Nezara viridula*, respectively, suppress efficiently plant defoliation. Additionally, these products indicated that beneficial species even closely relate species that are not harmed [63].

The *in vitro* transcription and the *in vivo* syntheses are basically the two nonchemical sources of pure dsRNA with potential for mass production. Both strategies are based on annealing of two single-stranded RNAs (ssRNAs) enzymatically synthetized. Therefore, the annealing of ssRNAs may be performed *in vitro* [18, 19, 41, 57] or *in vivo* using bacterial cells deficient of enzyme RNase III that degrades dsRNAs [35, 64, 65]; both approaches have advantages and disadvantages (**Table 1**). For example, there are possible hybridizations of two complementary ssRNA molecules that often result in a low final production of the correct and fully dsRNA duplexes. Moreover, the *in vivo* production may contain bacterial homologous DNA molecules that will affect RNA quality and its applicability.

In the last few years, we have experienced an ever-growing interest in the market for dsRNA that has pushed long-established companies and startups toward better production, cost-efficient, and stable delivery systems. In instance, the cost to produce 1 g of dsRNA (100 up to 800 pb) has dropped from $12,500 USD in 2008 to $100 USD in 2016, and to less than $60 USD today (July 2018) (http://www.agrorna.com/sub_05.html). The agroRNA [67] produces bulk amounts of dsRNA that could be used in agriculture; however, it is worth noting that naked dsRNA as sold by agroRNA needs to be formulated if the objective is a long-lasting

Approach	Cost	Purification	Labor demand	Mass production
In vivo	High	Hard	High	Possible
In vitro	Moderate	Easy	Medium	Maybe

*References: http://www.agrorna.com/ [9, 66].

Table 1. Common strategies* for mass production of dsRNA with pros and cons.

crop protection; otherwise, the dsRNAs will last only a few days. For crop protection, dsRNA does not need to be as pure as for medical application; however, at least for gene silencing in insects, the efficacy of dsRNA increased using purified RNA.

Considering the rapid half-life of dsRNA mainly regulated due to action of RNases and sunlight in the hostile environment, a biotechnology company RNAagri (former APSE) developed a technology "Apse RNA Containers" (ARCs) that allows the mass production of encapsulated ready-to-spray dsRNA with costs near $1 USD per 1 g [68]. In brief, this technology is based on plasmids engineered to produce naturally occurring proteins such as capsids that are cotransformed with another plasmid coding for the target dsRNA with a sequence called the "packing site." The proteins produced by bacteria self-assemble around RNAs, resulting in RNA protected and resistant to environmental hostile conditions. For long-lasting crop protection with exogenous applications, the dsRNAs should be protected with coating of nanoparticles, liposomes, or polymers, which will increase the efficacy by reducing dsRNA degradation [9].

Alternatively to pure dsRNA, the *Escherichia coli* [HT115(DE3)] strain can be used to produce large quantities of dsRNA. The crude extracts of bacterially expressed dsRNA can be sprayed on crops to protect against pest insects and plant pathogens [9, 10, 35]. Also, symbionts have shown to be a promising dsRNA delivery method [69]. These naturally occurring organisms such as virus/bacteria can be engineered to generate a symbiont-mediated RNAi system to continue produce dsRNA in the host. In perennial crops, there is a risk that the viral/bacterial genome could lose the dsRNA construct and revert to the wild type, while for annual crops, the area could be treated once and then deliver dsRNA during the entire production season.

The virus-induced gene silencing (VIGS) has also a great potential [70–72] to transiently silence target genes of insects or pathogens on host plants. Therefore, if an insect or pathogen-specific RNAi inducer sequence is introduced into an engineered plant virus, siRNAs specific for insect/pathogen targets will be produced upon plant infection [18, 73].

5. Postharvest protection using nontransformative RNAi

Yearly, vegetables, grains, flowers, and fresh fruits are damaged by microbial pathogens and insects. Sprays of dsRNA may also be efficient on postharvest products [19] to protect them during processing, transportation, and storage. Indeed, spraying *B. cinerea* dicer-like1/2 dsRNAs or sRNAs on the surface of fruits, vegetables, and flowers significantly inhibits gray mold diseases. Sprays of regular fungicides/insecticides commonly control insects and microbial pathogens attacking postharvest products, but sometimes these left residues on food. Also, mycotoxins, which are considered carcinogenic, are produced by fungal pathogens such as *Aspergillus* and *Fusarium* while proliferating on postharvest products. Sprays of dsRNA may also be used to control postharvest pest insects and pathogens as a new generation of sustainable and environmentally friendly products. It is worth to remind that postharvest products are not exposed to severe environment conditions such as sunlight, which contributes to reduced dsRNA degradation and long-lasting protection of postharvest products.

6. Other applications

RNAi naturally protects the cell from invasive viruses. Therefore, beyond the application of dsRNA sprays for pest and pathogen control, there is also a potential for the protection of beneficial insects such as bees from viral diseases. For example, the Israeli acute paralysis virus (IAPV) [74] is a single-stranded RNA virus in the family Dicistroviridae that increases bee mortality. The ingestion of dsRNAs from two regions of the IAPV genome protected bees from subsequent IAPV infection. The success of this experiment has encouraged field trials [75]. Large-scale field trials tested the efficiency of a dsRNA product, Rembee™ (Beeologics, LLC, Miami, FL, USA), in protecting honeybees from IAPV infection. The result was twice as many bees in the dsRNA-treated hives when compared to untreated hives. Additionally, dsRNA-treated hives produced threefold more honey than the untreated hives infected with IAPV. Similar results are also observed. A similar result was observed in bumblebees (*Bombus terrestris*) upon feeding of IAPV virus-specific dsRNAs that rescued the workers from mortality [76]. Also RNAi was efficient against the internal microsporidian parasites *Nosema apis* and *Nosema ceranae* [77] as well as Varroa mite *Varroa destructor* [78] and other mites [15], thus improving the honeybee health.

7. Conclusions

Crop protection against pathogens and pest insects relies mostly on the widespread use of chemical pesticides that are applied to the environment in large amounts yearly; some of these chemicals are in use for almost half a century. Therefore, there is a need for novel tools more sustainable and less detrimental to the environment. Therefore, scientists have harnessed RNAi to turn off genes that they are studying. RNAi through nontransformative strategies will demand mass production of dsRNA, efficient delivery methods, and methods to validate its environmental stability.

A large number of studies have demonstrated the feasibility and efficacy of RNAi-based approaches, and some transgenic plants have been approved for commercialization and release [38, 39, 79, 80]. However, unlike these strategies, which depend on plant transformation, the spray of dsRNA externally realizes crop protection without changing the plant DNA. The dsRNA-containing end-use products, nevertheless, will be differently regulated when compared to transgenic plants such as *Bacillus thuringiensis* crops. Moreover, chemical compounds act through a structure-dependent mechanism, and dsRNA acts though a tailored species-specific sequence. Clearly, the dsRNA has more changes to act only against the target species. Also, multiple target genes could be silenced simultaneously by fusing dsRNA sequences to generate a pyramidic plant protection approach, without any modification of the plant genome.

It is worth to remind that a specific dsRNA exerts its mode of action throughout entire sequence length by generating a large pool of target-specific siRNAs [29, 30, 32]. This large pool of siRNAs for a single target increases target specificity and largely reduces evolution of mutations and resistance in the targeted organism. Indeed, the dsRNA is designed to match a long nucleotide sequences in the target organism (i.e., insects, pathogens, or viruses). The effectiveness of a long dsRNA will remain even when parts of this sequence mutate. So that it is believed that it is unlike to face resistance evolution that commonly makes a chemical pesticide ineffective. Resistance development toward RNAi has not been documented in insects and fungi, but as a famous artist says, *"life finds a way,"* these organisms have a great phenotypic and genetic plasticity and relatively short life cycle contributing for that some individuals/strains could be more or less sensitive to RNAi. For example, issues such as malfunction of dsRNA uptake or nuclease upregulation and/or processing dsRNA and systemic spread of RNAi signaling could stop the initiation and spread of RNAi response [45]. At least for arthropod species as recently reviewed [45], the potential degradation of dsRNA prior to ingestion, breakdown by nucleases in saliva and/or in the gastrointestinal tract, degradation of dsRNA in the hemolymph, and/or transport mechanisms of dsRNA within the organism are some of several barriers to physiological exposure that may lead to resistance.

The sprayed dsRNAs, different from regular pesticides, are biocompatible compounds as they occur naturally in the nature as well as inside/outside body of organisms and in food. The dsRNA ultimately is a regular RNA molecule that enters naturally within plants and other organisms. These molecules are subject of pathways from RNAi silencing mechanism, converted into siRNA and finally degraded by natural cell processes. In water and soil, dsRNAs are rapidly degraded as regular RNA molecules do [81], so unlike to left considerably novel residues in food products.

New genomic tools will allow the development of technologies such as dsRNA sprays that increase crop resistance against insects, pathogens, and viruses; these could even replace chemical pesticides in some applications.

Acknowledgements

The authors acknowledge support over the years for their RNAi-related research from the National Council for Scientific and Technological Development (CNPq) and Coordination for the Improvement of Higher Education Personnel (CAPES) in Brazil and from the Foundation Research-Flanders (FWO-Vlaanderen) and the Special Research Fund of Ghent University (BOF-UGent) in Belgium.

Author details

Deise Cagliari[1], Ericmar Avila dos Santos[1], Naymã Dias[1], Guy Smagghe[2] and Moises Zotti[1]*

*Address all correspondence to: moises.zotti@ufpel.edu.br

1 Department of Crop Protection, Molecular Entomology, Federal University of Pelotas, Pelotas, Brazil

2 Department of Plants and Crops, Faculty of Bioscience Engineering, Ghent University, Ghent, Belgium

References

[1] Oerke E-C. Crop losses to pests. The Journal of Agricultural Science. 2006;**144**(1):31

[2] Hollomon DW. Do we have the tools to manage resistance in the future? Pest Management Science. 2012;**68**(2):149-154

[3] Gatehouse AMR, Ferry N, Edwards MG, Bell HA. Insect-resistant biotech crops and their impacts on beneficial arthropods. Philosophical Transactions of the Royal Society B: Biological Sciences. 2011;**366**(1569):1438-1452

[4] Fire A, Albertson D, Harrison SW, Moerman DG. Production of antisense RNA leads to effective and specific inhibition of gene expression in C. Elegans muscle. Development. 1991;**113**(2):503-514

[5] Fire A, Xu S, Montgomery MK, Kostas SA, Driver SE, Mello CC. Potent and specific genetic interference by double-stranded RNA in *Caenorhabditis elegans*. Nature. 1998; **391**(6669):806-811

[6] Gordon KHJ, Waterhouse PM. RNAi for insect-proof plants. Nature Biotechnology. 2007; **25**(11):1231-1232

[7] Price DRG, Gatehouse JA. RNAi-mediated crop protection against insects. Trends in Biotechnology. 2008;**26**(7):393-400

[8] Huvenne H, Smagghe G. Mechanisms of dsRNA uptake in insects and potential of RNAi for pest control : A review. Journal of Insect Physiology. 2010;**56**(3):227-235

[9] Joga MR, Zotti MJ, Smagghe G, Christiaens O. RNAi efficiency, systemic properties, and novel delivery methods for pest insect control: What we know so far. Frontiers in Physiology. 2016;**7**(November):553

[10] San Miguel K, Scott JG. The next generation of insecticides: DsRNA is stable as a foliar-applied insecticide. Pest Management Science. 2016;**72**(4):801-809

[11] Andrade EC, Hunter WB. RNA interference – natural gene-based technology for highly specific pest control (HiSPeC). In: Abdurakhmonov IY, editor. RNA Interference. Rijeka: InTech; 2016. pp. 391-409

[12] Zotti M, dos Santos EA, Cagliari D, Christiaens O, Taning CNT, Smagghe G. RNAi technology in crop protection against arthropod pests, pathogens and nematodes. Pest Management Science. 2018;**74**(6):1239-1250

[13] Wu K, Hoy MA. Clathrin heavy chain is important for viability, oviposition, embryogenesis and, possibly, systemic RNAi response in the predatory mite *Metaseiulus occidentalis*. PLoS One. 2014;**9**(10):e110874

[14] Kwon DH, Park JH, Ashok PA, Lee U, Lee SH. Screening of target genes for RNAi in *Tetranychus urticae* and RNAi toxicity enhancement by chimeric genes. Pesticide Biochemistry and Physiology. 2016;**130**:1-7

[15] Niu J, Shen G, Christiaens O, Smagghe G, He L, Wang J. Beyond insects: Current status, achievements and future perspectives of RNAi in mite pests. Pest Management Science. 2018. DOI: 10.1002/ps.5071

[16] de la Fuente J, Kocan KM, Almazán C, Blouin EF. RNA interference for the study and genetic manipulation of ticks. Trends in Parasitology. 2007;**23**(9):427-433

[17] Koch A, Kumar N, Weber L, Keller H, Imani J, Kogel K-H. Host-induced gene silencing of cytochrome P450 lanosterol C14-demethylase-encoding genes confers strong resistance to *Fusarium* species. Proceedings of the National Academy of Sciences. 2013;**110**(48):19324-19329

[18] Koch A, Biedenkopf D, Furch A, Weber L, Rossbach O, Abdellatef E, et al. An RNAi-based control of *Fusarium graminearum* infections through spraying of long dsRNAs involves a plant passage and is controlled by the fungal silencing machinery. PLoS Pathogens. 2016;**12**(10):e1005901

[19] Wang M, Weiberg A, Lin F-M, Thomma BPHJ, Huang H-D, Jin H. Bidirectional cross-kingdom RNAi and fungal uptake of external RNAs confer plant protection. Nature Plants. 2016;**2**(10):16151

[20] Fu D-Q, Zhu B-Z, Zhu H-L, Jiang W-B, Luo Y-B. Virus-induced gene silencing in tomato fruit. The Plant Journal. 2005;**43**(2):299-308

[21] Jahan SN, Åsman AKM, Corcoran P, Fogelqvist J, Vetukuri RR, Dixelius C. Plant-mediated gene silencing restricts growth of the potato late blight pathogen *Phytophthora infestans*. Journal of Experimental Botany. 2015;**66**(9):2785-2794

[22] Duan C-G, Wang C-H, Guo H-S. Application of RNA silencing to plant disease resistance. Silence. 2012;**3**(1):5

[23] Tabassum B, Ahmad I, Aslam U, Husnai T. How RNA interference combat viruses in plants. In: Meroni G, Petrera F, editors. Functional Genomics. Rijeka: InTech; 2012. pp. 113-130

[24] Shaner DL, Beckie HJ. The future for weed control and technology. Pest Management Science. 2014;**70**(9):1329-1339

[25] Bond DM, Baulcombe DC. Epigenetic transitions leading to heritable, RNA-mediated de novo silencing in Arabidopsis thaliana. Proceedings of the National Academy of Sciences. 2015;**112**(3):201413053

[26] Baum JA, Roberts JK. Chapter Five - Progress Towards RNAi-Mediated Insect Pest Management. In: Dhadialla TS, Gill IP, editors. Insect Midgut and Insecticidal Proteins. Vol. 47. Academic Press; 2014. pp. 249-295

[27] Mao J, Zeng F. Plant-mediated RNAi of a gap gene-enhanced tobacco tolerance against the *Myzus persicae*. Transgenic Research. 2014;**23**(1):145-152

[28] Hunter WB, Glick E, Paldi N, Bextine BR. Advances in RNA interference: dsRNA treatment in trees and grapevines for insect pest suppression. South West Entomology. 2012;**37**(1):85-87

[29] Preall JB, Sontheimer EJ. RNAi: RISC gets loaded. Cell. 2005;**123**(4):543-545

[30] Agrawal N, Dasaradhi PVN, Mohmmed A, Malhotra P, Bhatnagar RK, Mukherjee SK. RNA interference: Biology, mechanism, and applications. Microbiology and Molecular Biology Reviews. 2003;**67**(4):657-685

[31] Ghildiyal M, Zamore PD. Small silencing RNAs: An expanding universe. Nature Reviews. Genetics. 2009;**10**(2):94-108

[32] Carthew RW, Sontheimer EJ. Origins and Mechanisms of miRNAs and siRNAs. Cell. 2009;**136**(4):642-655

[33] Wilson RC, Doudna JA. Molecular mechanisms of RNA interference. Annual Review of Biophysics. 2013;**42**(1):217-239

[34] Borges F, Martienssen RA. The expanding world of small RNAs in plants. Nature Reviews Molecular Cell Biology. 2015;**16**(12):727-741

[35] Tenllado F, Martínez-García B, Vargas M, Díaz-Ruíz JR. Crude extracts of bacterially expressed dsRNA can be used to protect plants against virus infections. BMC Biotechnology. 2003;**3**(1):3

[36] Baum JA, Bogaert T, Clinton W, Heck GR, Feldmann P, Ilagan O, et al. Control of coleopteran insect pests through RNA interference. Nature Biotechnol. 2007;**25**(11):1322-1326

[37] Mao Y-B, Cai W-J, Wang J-W, Hong G-J, Tao X-Y, Wang L-J, et al. Silencing a cotton bollworm P450 monooxygenase gene by plant-mediated RNAi impairs larval tolerance of gossypol. Nature Biotechnology. 2007;**25**(11):1307-1313

[38] Head GP, Carroll MW, Evans SP, Rule DM, Willse AR, Clark TL, et al. Evaluation of SmartStax and SmartStax PRO maize against western corn rootworm and northern corn rootworm: Efficacy and resistance management. Pest Management Science. 2017;**73**(9): 1883-1899

[39] Gonsalves D, Street A, Ferreira S. Transgenic virus resistant papaya: From hope to reality for controlling papaya Ringspot virus in Hawaii. APSnet. 2004;(July):12 Online. DOI: 10.1094/APSnetFeature-2004-0704

[40] Khalid A, Zhang Q, Yasir M, Li F. Small RNA based genetic engineering for plant viral resistance: Application in crop protection. Frontiers in Microbiology. 2017;**8**(January):1-11

[41] Tenllado F, Díaz-Ruíz JR. Double-stranded RNA-mediated interference with plant virus infection. Journal of Virology. 2001;**75**(24):12288-12297

[42] Youssef RM, Kim KH, Haroon SA, Matthews BF. Post-transcriptional gene silencing of the gene encoding aldolase from soybean cyst nematode by transformed soybean roots. Experimental Parasitology. 2013;**134**(2):266-274

[43] Yang Y, Jittayasothorn Y, Chronis D, Wang X, Cousins P, Zhong GY. Molecular characteristics and efficacy of 16D10 siRNAs in inhibiting root-knot nematode infection in transgenic grape hairy roots. PLoS One. 2013;**8**(7):e69463

[44] Zotti M, dos Santos EA, Cagliari D, Christiaens O, Taning CNT, Smagghe G. RNA interference technology in crop protection against arthropod pests, pathogens and nematodes. Pest Management Science. 2018;**74**(6):1239-1250

[45] Christiaens O, Dzhambazova T, Kostov K, Arpaia S, Joga MR, Urru I, et al. Literature review of baseline information to support the risk assessment of RNAi-based GM plants. EFSA Support Publications. Wiley; 2018;**15**(5)

[46] Hunter WB, Glick E, Paldi N, Bextine BR. Advances in RNA interference: dsRNA treatment in trees and grapevines for insect pest suppression. South West Entomology. 2012;**37**(1):85-87

[47] Melnyk CW, Molnar A, Baulcombe DC. Intercellular and systemic movement of RNA silencing signals. The EMBO Journal. 2011;**30**(17):3553-3563

[48] Kupferschmidt K. A lethal dose of RNA. Science (80-). 2013;**341**(6147):732-733

[49] US EPA - Environment Protection Agency, RNAi Technology as a Pesticide: Problem Formulation for Human Health and Ecological Risk Assessment. 2013. http://www.thecre.com/premium/wp-content/uploads/2012/04/RNAi-White-Paper.pdf [acessed 05 may 2018]

[50] US EPA - Environment Protection Agency, RNAi Technology as a Pesticide: Problem Formulation for Human Health and Ecological Risk Assessment. 2014. http://www.epa.gov/sites/production/files/2015-06/documents/012814minutes.pdf [acessed 05 June 2018]

[51] Zotti MJ, Smagghe G. RNAi technology for insect management and protection of beneficial insects from diseases: Lessons, challenges and risk assessments. Neotropical Entomology. 2015;**44**(3):197-213

[52] US EPA - Environment Protection Agency, RNAi Technology: Human Health and Ecological Risk Assessments for SmartStax PRO. (2016). https://www.epa.gov/sites/production/files/2016-12/documents/rnai_sap_sept_2016_final_minutes.pdf [acessed 10 June 2018]

[53] Li H, Guan R, Guo H, Miao X. New insights into an RNAi approach for plant defence against piercing-sucking and stem-borer insect pests. Plant, Cell and Environment. 2015; **38**(11):2277-2285

[54] Tenllado F, Llave C, Díaz-Ruíz JR. RNA interference as a new biotechnological tool for the control of virus diseases in plants. Virus Research. 2004;**102**(1):85-96

[55] Mitter N, Worrall EA, Robinson KE, Li P, Jain RG, Taochy C. Clay nanosheets for topical delivery of RNAi for sustained protection against plant viruses. Nature Plants. 2017;**3**:16207

[56] Mitter N, Worrall EA, Robinson KE, Xu ZP, Carroll BJ. Induction of virus resistance by exogenous application of double-stranded RNA. Current Opinion in Virology. 2017; **26**:49-55

[57] Konakalla NC, Kaldis A, Berbati M, Masarapu H, Voloudakis AE. Exogenous application of double-stranded RNA molecules from TMV p126 and CP genes confers resistance against TMV in tobacco. Planta. 2016;**244**(4):961-969

[58] Dang Y, Yang Q, Xue Z, Liu Y. RNA interference in fungi: Pathways, functions, and applications. Eukaryotic Cell. 2011;**10**(9):1148-1155

[59] Whangbo JS, Hunter CP. Environmental RNA interference. Trends in Genetics. 2008;**24**(6): 297-305

[60] Mitter N, Worrall EA, Robinson KE, Li P, Jain RG, Taochy C, et al. Induction of virus resistance by exogenous application of double-stranded RNA. Nature Plants. 2017;**16207** (January)

[61] Saleh M, Van Rij RP, Hekele A, Gillis A, Foley E, Farrell PHO, et al. The endocytic pathway mediates cell entry of dsRNA to induce RNAi silencing. Nature Cell Biology. 2006; **8**(8):793-802

[62] Ivashuta S, Zhang Y, Wiggins BE, Ramaseshadri P, Segers GC, Johnson S, et al. Environmental RNAi in herbivorous insects. RNA. 2015;**21**(5):1-11

[63] Plaetinck G, RNA-Based Biocontrols: een nieuwe technologie voor insectbestrijding. 2017. Avaliable from: https://www.ctgb.nl/binaries/ctgb/documenten/publicatie/2017/06/15/presentaties-relatiedag-2017/grote-zaal-gew-sessie-c-geert-plaetinck.pdf

[64] Voloudakis AE, Holeva MC, Sarin PS, Bamford DH, Vargas MM, Poranen M, Tenllado F. Efficient Double-Stranded RNA Production Methods for Utilization in Plant Virus Control. In: Uyeda I, Masuta C, editors. Plant Virology Protocols. Methods in Molecular Biology (Methods and Protocols). Vol. 1236. New York, NY: Humana Press; 2015. pp. 255-274

[65] Prentice K, Pertry I, Christiaens O, Bauters L, Bailey A, Niblett C, et al. Transcriptome analysis and systemic RNAi response in the African sweetpotato weevil (*Cylas puncticollis*, Coleoptera, *Brentidae*). PLoS One. 2015;**10**(1):1-18

[66] Niehl A, Soininen M, Poranen MM, Heinlein M. Synthetic biology approach for plant protection using dsRNA. Plant Biotechnology Journal. 2018:1-9. DOI: 10.1111/pbi.12904

[67] AgroRNA. 2018. [Online]. Available: http://www.agrorna.com/sub_05.html [12 May 2018]

[68] APSE – The manufacturing cost leaders in RNA. 2017. [Online]. Available: http://www.apsellc.com/ [12 July 2018]

[69] Whitten MM, Facey PD, Del Sol R, Evans MC, Mitchell JJ, Bodger OG, et al. Symbiont-mediated RNA interference in insects. Proceedings of the Royal Society B. 2016;**283**(1825): 20160042

[70] Lu R, Martin-Hernandez AM, Peart JR, Malcuit I, Baulcombe DC. Virus-induced gene silencing in plants. Methods. 2003;**30**(4):296-303

[71] Kolliopoulou A, Taning CNT, Smagghe G, Swevers L. Viral delivery of dsRNA for control of insect agricultural pests and vectors of human disease: Prospects and challenges. Frontiers in Physiology. 2017;**8**(June):1-24

[72] Taning CNT, Christiaens O, Li X, Swevers L, Casteels H, Maes M, et al. Engineered flock house virus for targeted gene suppression through RNAi in fruit flies (*Drosophila melanogaster*) in vitro and in vivo. Frontiers in Physiology. 2018;**9**(July):1-13

[73] Nandety RS, Kuo YW, Nouri S, Falk BW. Emerging strategies for RNA interference (RNAI) applications in insects. Bioengineered. Bugs. 2015;**6**(1):8-19

[74] Maori E, Paldi N, Shafir S, Kalev H, Tsur E, Glick E, et al. IAPV, a bee-affecting virus associated with colony collapse disorder can be silenced by dsRNA ingestion. Insect Molecular Biology. 2009;**18**(1):55-60

[75] Hunter W, Ellis J, Vanengelsdorp D, Hayes J, Westervelt D, Glick E, et al. Large-scale field application of RNAi technology reducing Israeli acute paralysis virus disease in honey bees (*Apis mellifera*, hymenoptera: Apidae). PLoS Pathogens. 2010;**6**(12):1-10

[76] Piot N, Snoeck S, Vanlede M, Smagghe G, Meeus I. The effect of oral administration of dsRNA on viral replication and mortality in *Bombus terrestris*. Viruses. 2015;**7**(6):3172-3185

[77] Paldi N, Glick E, Oliva M, Zilberberg Y, Aubin L, Pettis J, et al. Effective gene silencing in a microsporidian parasite associated with honeybee (*Apis mellifera*) colony declines. Applied and Environmental Microbiology. 2010;**76**(17):5960-5964

[78] Garbian Y, Maori E, Kalev H, Shafir S, Sela I. Bidirectional transfer of RNAi between honey bee and *Varroa destructor*: Varroa gene silencing reduces *Varroa* population. PLoS Pathogens. 2012;**8**(12):e1003035

[79] Dolgov S, Mikhaylov R, Serova T, Shulga O, Firsov A. Pathogen-derived methods for improving resistance of transgenic plums (*Prunus domestica* L.) for plum pox virus infection. 21st International Confererence on Viruses and Other Graft Transmissible Diseases of Fruit Crops. 2010;**6**(21):133-140

[80] Scorza R, Callahan A, Dardick C, Ravelonandro M, Polak J, Malinowski T, et al. Genetic engineering of plum pox virus resistance: 'HoneySweet' plum-from concept to product. Plant Cell, Tissue and Organ Culture. 2013;**115**(1):1-12

[81] Dubelman S, Fischer J, Zapata F, Huizinga K, Jiang C, Uffman J, et al. Environmental fate of double-stranded RNA in agricultural soils. PLoS One. 2014;**9**(3):1-7

Section 3

Novel Gene Silencing Methodologies

Chapter 5

Strand Displacement Amplification for Multiplex Detection of Nucleic Acids

Lingwen Zeng, Omar Mukama, Xuewen Lu,
Shilin Cao and Donghai Lin

Additional information is available at the end of the chapter

http://dx.doi.org/10.5772/intechopen.80687

Abstract

The identification of various targets such as bacteria, viruses, and other cells remains a prerequisite for point-of-care diagnostics and biotechnological applications. Nucleic acids, as encoding information for all forms of life, are excellent biomarkers for detecting pathogens, hereditary diseases, and cancers. To date, many techniques have been developed to detect nucleic acids. However, most of them are based on polymerase chain reaction (PCR) technology. These methods are sensitive and robust, but they require expensive instruments and trained personnel. DNA strand displacement amplification is carried out under isothermal conditions and therefore does not need expensive instruments. It is simple, fast, sensitive, specific, and inexpensive. In this chapter, we introduce the principles, methods, and updated applications of DNA strand displacement technology in the detection of infectious diseases. We also discuss how robust, sensitive, and specific nucleic acid detection could be obtained when combined with the novel CRISPR/Cas system.

Keywords: nucleic acids, isothermal amplification, strand displacement, CRISPR/Cas, multiplex detection

1. Introduction

To date, nucleic acids have been used not only for biological studies but also as powerful biomarkers for clinical diagnosis, agriculture, forensic science, and so on. PCR is a well-known molecular biology tool for the amplification of target sequences. In PCR, DNA amplification relies on heating and cooling of nucleic acids followed by hybridization. It can efficiently amplify target sequences within a few hours in three temperature-dependent steps: initiation, annealing, and elongation. However, PCR requires thermocyclers for reaction temperature adjustment and trained personnel, which hinders its usage in resource-limited settings; and additionally, it has mispriming and sometimes inadequate template amplification. Therefore, the development of simple and inexpensive methods for nucleic acids amplification and detection is important for on-site inspections.

Whilst several isothermal amplification platforms, such as nucleic acid sequence based amplification (NASBA) [1], strand displacement amplification (SDA) [2–5], loop-mediated isothermal amplification (LAMP) [6], rolling circle amplification (RCA) [7], recombinase polymerase amplification (RPA) [8], and Helicase dependent Isothermal DNA Amplification (HAD) [9, 10] have been developed. These amplification platforms can achieve linear or exponential dsDNA accumulation, and some of which can be purchased as kits and integrated in portable devices [5], so no expensive instruments are needed, but there are still challenges in multiplexing, primer design, and stringency in experimental design. In this chapter, we describe the development and current directions of SDA in detail. Prospects in analysis using fluorescence, colorimetry, and lateral flow biosensors are also discussed.

Moreover, CRISPR-Cas system is also currently exploited for the detection of nucleic acids. For instance, some CRISPR-Cas proteins have been found to exhibit collateral cleavage of target nucleic acids and any nonspecific single-stranded nucleic acids in the solution. Therefore, if the latter is labeled with a fluorescent or a specific antibody recognized molecule, detectable signal can be generated [11–13]. This combination of isothermal amplification and various CRISPR-Cas-based signal readouts is simple, fast, specific, and sensitive and thus can elevate the specificity of nucleic acid diagnosis. In addition, CRISPR-Cas-based diagnosis can be multiplexed to provide another convergent evolution and convenient point-of-care detection of nucleic acids in low cost.

2. Strand displacement amplification (SDA)

SDA is carried out under isothermal condition. It is inspired from normal physiological RNA transcription and DNA replication, which occurs at a constant temperature. Over the past 2 decades, SDA has been widely used as an alternative to PCR for the detection of pathogens [14, 15], hereditary diseases [16], and cancers [17–19]. Moreover, SDA amplified nucleic acids can be multiplexed and readily provide optical and visual readouts [14, 20, 21]. In a typical SDA, two pairs of primers are designed to specifically recognize two regions of a target sequence. One pair is bumper primers designed as standard PCR primers, and another pair is SDA primers, which bind immediately next to the bumper primers at the target sequences. In addition, a HincII restriction enzyme and an exonuclease deficient (exo^- Klenow) polymerase are added. The reaction mixture is incubated in a single constant temperature of 37°C. In this reaction, the *Hinc*II cleaves at the recognition site of the phosphorothioate (modified substrate, dATPαS) of the DNA probe, and the *exo*$^-$ Klenow initiates the replication of the sequence. Subsequently, the exponential reaction starts with the primer-triggered repeated cycle of nicking, extension, and strand displacement. This amplification is accelerated by additional primers franking the inner region of the target sequence, and this reaction exhibits a single and double nicking site cycle (**Figure 1**). The final new product chain yield can reach 10^7-fold amplification within 2 h [2, 20]. However, unlike the original method of cutting double-stranded sequences using restriction enzymes, the modified SDA uses nicking endonucleases (engineered restriction enzymes) such as Nt.BsmAI, Nb.BsmI, Nb.BsrDI, Nt.BspQI, Nb.BtsI, Nt.AlwI, Nt.BbvCI, and Nt.BstNBI (**Table 1**) to enhance the site-specific cleavage accuracy of target sequences and do not require modified dNTPs such as dATPαS at the cleavage site.

These endonucleases effectively create a nick for Klenow fragment or *Bst* polymerase to initiate a new strand replication and displace the downstream strand. The improved SDA exhibits an enhanced exponential amplification at 37–55°C, with 10^9-fold amplified DNA in <30 min [3]. The amplified nucleic acid products can be detected by photometry (turbidity), electrophoresis, SYBR Green's DNA-insertion dye, cross-flow text of a sequence-specific hybridization capture probe, or visual inspection of white precipitate. As shown in **Figure 1**, DNA double-strand is denatured, and primers (S1, S2, B1, and B2) bind to a specific DNA polymerase such as exo⁻ Klenow or Bst and then extend through the strand displacement activity. Upon the formation of strand containing the nicking site (linear amplification), the nicking enzyme cleave it, and the DNA polymerase primes initiate a new round of replication (1st cycle). The exponential amplification continues with a cycle of single and double-nicking, extension, and displacement cycles, producing a targeting sequence (SDA product).

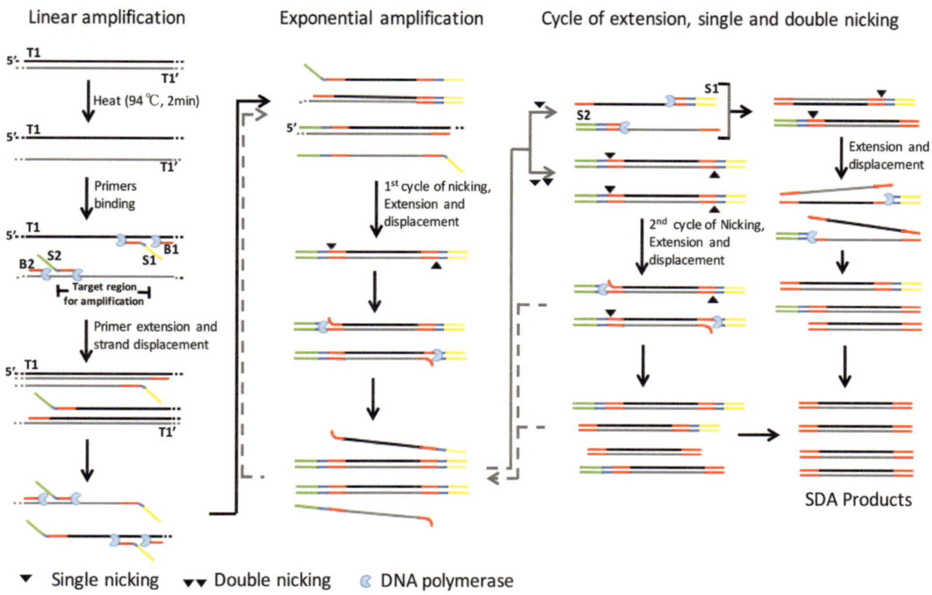

Figure 1. Schematic illustration of strand displacement isothermal amplification principle. First, double strand DNA is heat denatured for primer binding. The SDA primers (S1 and S2) contain recognition sequence for nicking endonuclease (green and yellow), a linker (blue), and sequence complementary to a target sequence (red). Bumper primers (B1 and B2) are located upstream of the SDA primers (red) and are complementary to the target sequence (black and gray). These primers bind to target sequence and extend by specific DNA polymerase such as exo⁻ Klenow or Bst with strand displacement activity. Upon formation of strands harboring a nicking site (linear amplification), the nicking enzyme nicks them, and the DNA polymerase primes a new round of replication (first cycle). Exponential amplification of the target sequence starts by cycle of single and double nicking, extension, and displacement.

Target	NEases	Template	Sample	DNA polymerase	Time (min)	Sensitivity	Detection method	Refs.
Singlex								
Salmonella spp.	Nt.BbvCI, b.Bpu10I	DNA aptamer	Bacteria strains, spiked milk	Exo^- Klenow, Bsm	30	1–60 CFU/ml	Lateral flow, G-quadruplex	[15, 22]
Hepatitis	Nt.BstNBI	DNA	HBV positive serum	Bst 2.0	30	2.5×10^4 copies	Electrophoresis and real-time fluorescence	[23]
E. Coli O157:H7	Nt.BbvCI	DNA aptamer	Bacteria strains, spiked milk	Exo^- Klenow	30	10 CFU/ml	Lateral flow	[24]
Mycobacterium (singlex)	*Hinc*II-*Eco*RI(Gl11)	DNA	DNA-spiked samples	Exo^- Klenow	120	<5 genome copies	Fluorescence polarization	[25]
Human papilloma virus	Nt.BsmAI	DNA	clinical samples and cell lines	Exo^- Klenow and phi29	30	0.1 pM–1 nM	Real-time fluorescence	[26]
HIV	BsoBI	RNA	RNA	Bst	55	250 copies	Fluorescence and flow cytometry	[27]
Bacillus cereus	-	gDNA	Bacteria strains, spiked human DNA	Exo^- Klenow and phi29	120	From 1 pg	NGS and real-time fluorescence	[28]
Simian Virus 40	-	DNA		Exo^- Klenow	40	1–250 pM	G-quadruplex	[21]
Heavy metals (e.g., Hg^{2+})	Nt.AlwI	DNA	Spiked tap water	Exo^- Klenow	30	2.95	Real-time fluorescence	[29]
Toxins (e.g., aflatoxin)	Nb.BbvCI	DNA	Skimmed milk sample	Exo^- Klenow	30	17–18 ng/kg	G-quadruplex fluorescence	[30]
$VEGF_{165}$	Nb.BbvCI	DNA aptamer	Spiked human serum	Bst	-	5–400 pg/ml	Fluorescence	[31]
Breast, prostate	Nt.AlwI	DNA	Spiked human serum	Exo^- Klenow	30	0.47 U/L	Real-time fluorescence, Sybr Green I	[32]
K-Ras	Nt.BbvCI	DNA	Cell lines	Exo^- Klenow	120	4 pM	Colorimetric and electrochemical immunosensing	[33]
MTase	Nb.BbvCI	DNA	Cell lines, spiked Dam MTase human serum	Exo^- Klenow	30	0.063 U/mL	G-quadruplex fluorescence	[34]

http://dx.doi.org/10.5772/intechopen.80687

Target	NEases	Template	Sample	DNA polymerase	Time (min)	Sensitivity	Detection method	Refs.
p53	-	DNA	Mutant *p53* DNA	Exo^- Klenow	25	250 pmol/l	G-quadruplex fluorescence, Sybr Green I	[35]
miRNAs	Nt.AlwI	miRNA	miRNA, spiked serum	Exo^- Klenow	90	16 zmol	Electrophoresis and real-time fluorescence	[18]
Stem cells	Nt.BbvCI	DNA aptamer	Stem cell lines	Exo^- Klenow	30	19 cells	Lateral flow	[36]
Cocaine	-	DNA	Spiked human serum and complex media	Exo^- Klenow	60	2 nM	Electrophoresis, real-time fluorescence, SYBR Green I	[37]
GMOs and mutagens	Nt.*Bsm*AI	RNA	Rice leaves	phi29	150	0.14 fM	Electrochemiluminescence	[38]
Multiplex								
Mycobacterium species	*Hinc*II	DNA	DNA, human placental DNA	Exo^- Klenow	120	<5 genome copies	Fluorescence polarization	[20]
Neisseria gonorrhoeae and *Chlamydia trachomatis*	NA	DNA	Genital and urine samples	NA	60	75%	BD ProbeTec System-fluorescence reader	[14]
E. coli O157:H7 and its serotypes	BsoBI	DNA	Bovine, water and drinks	Bst polymerase	30	4.3 bacteria	Fluorescence polarization	[39]
Vibrio and *E. Coli* O157:H7	-	DNA	Bacteria strains, spiked serum	Bst 2.0	30	3.5 cells	Gel electrophoresis and lateral flow	[40]
MicroRNAs	Nt.BbvCI	miRNA	HepG2 cells, spiked lysates	Exo^- Klenow	90	5 pM	G-quadruplex fluorescence	[41]
S. aureus, engineered internal control sequences	Nt.BbvCI	Synthetic DNAs	DNA, simulated nasal matrix	Bst2.0WarmStart	<20	10–50 copies	Real-time fluorescence and lateral flow	[3]

NEases: nicking endonuclease, ↓: cut at 5′-3′ complementary strand, ↑: cut at 3′-5′ complementary strand, Nt: Nicking at top strand, Nb: Nicking at bottom strand, and MTase: DNA methyl transferase.

Table 1. Singlex and multiplex detection of nucleic acids using SDA-based assays.

2.1 Experimental procedures

2.1.1 Design of SDA primers

Primers are prerequisite for the initiation of nucleic acid amplification. SDA requires two pairs of primers, SDA primers (S1 and S2), and Bumper primers (B1 and B2). Bumper primers are similar to standard PCR forward and reverse primers for the identification of specific sites and amplification of a target DNA sequence. The B1 and B2 primers are 18–23 nucleotides designed based on the target strand from the 5′ end and a reverse complementary sequence of the 3′ end strand, respectively. However, the S1 and S2 primers are a pair of 5′ end-turned special primers. From 5′ to 3′, both primers contain a protecting 10–15 nucleotides, a nicking recognition sequence (~5 nucleotides), linkage sequence (~4 nucleotides), and then a 10–18 nucleotides complementary to the target sequence at the 3′ end immediately adjacent to a bumper primer (**Figure 1**).

2.1.2 Properties and choice of nicking endonuclease

Restriction endonucleases are well-known endonucleases that recognize and cleave palindromic DNA sequences. Nicking endonucleases (NEases), on the other hand, cleave one strand of a specific DNA sequence. Typically, homodimer restriction enzymes bind to two half sites of a specific palindromic sequence, that is, each monomer cut one strand. However, both the nicking endonucleases and one strand-cleaving restriction enzyme are heterodimers, allowing only single nicking or cleaving at the asymmetric recognition sequences. Through the genetic engineering of naturally occurring restriction enzymes, various nicking endonucleases, such as Nb.BbvCI and Nt.BbvCI, have been generated through modifications of the catalytic activity of the asymmetric amino acid sequences of the enzymes. BbvCI, a heterodimeric Type IIS endonuclease recognizing 7 bp of asymmetric DNA sequence, uses its R1 and R2 subunits at the catalytic sites to cleave bottom strand and top strand (..CC↓TCAGC.. and ..CCTCA↑GC..), respectively [3, 42]. The Nt.BbvCI is an engineered BbvCI with functional R2 and a missing R1 domain which can only cleave top strand (..CC↓TCAGC..) [42, 43], while Nb.BbvCI was engineered from BbvCI, with functional R1 and deficient R2, which can only cleave bottom strand (CCTCA↑GC..) [43]. However, other nicking endonucleases were generated through mutations, truncation, and domain swapping. These nicking endonucleases include bottom strand nickase such as Nt.AlwI, Nb.BsmI [44], Nb.BsrDI, Nt.BspQI [45], Nb.BtsI, and Nt.CviQII and top strand nickase such as Nt.CviPII [46–48]. For example, Nt.AlwI was engineered from the dimeric AlwI (dsDNA cleaving REase) to cleave only the top strand of the AlwI target sequence (..GGATCNNNNN↓N..). The Nt.AlwI monomer structure derives from the dimerization swapping with nonfunctional domain of Nt.BstNBI [49]. Thus, as shown in **Table 1**, the choice of nicking enzymes may depend on the preferred DNA polymerase and the desired type of reaction to achieve an efficient amplification.

2.1.3 Properties and choice of DNA polymerase

The combinations of nicking enzymes and DNA polymerases have great effect on the amplification efficiency. For example, among several nicking enzymes and DNA polymerases studied, Nt.BspQI coupled with Sequenase 2.0 polymerase showed a higher linear SDA amplification [47], and Nt.BstNBI coupled with Bst DNA polymerase showed a 10 times higher exponential amplification compared to other combinatorial NEases. The authors attributed this property to the enzymatic conformation and concentration, as higher or lower concentration could be ineffective for the SDA reaction [50]. DNA polymerase such as exo⁻ Klenow and Bst (Bst 2.0, Bst 2.0 WarmStart, and Bst 3.0) have good amplification performance and are good choices for SDA [3]. Although Exo⁻ Klenow exhibits excellent performance after binding to specific nicking enzymes like Nb.BbvCI, the amplification efficiency decreases by 5–100 folds when the target nucleic acid sequence increases by 50 base pairs [47]. Bst exhibits a similar limitation. To address the limitation of Exo⁻ Klenow and Bst, newly engineered DNA polymerases such as Bst 2.0 show higher efficiency, thermal stability, salt tolerance, and greater fidelity in SDA amplification. Xu et al. showed that Bst 2.0 polymerase highly prefers Nt.BbvCI rather than other conventional nicking enzymes, and this combination showed good results for the detection of viral, bacteria, and *BRCA1* gene sequences. However, various inhibitors can affect the activity of most polymerases. Fortunately, Bst 3.0 was designed to amplify both RNA and DNA with high activity even in the presence of amplification inhibitors.

Furthermore, to encounter mispriming occurring at lower temperatures and isothermal amplification stringency, Bst 2.0 WarmStart was engineered. A specific aptamer (unique oligonucleotide sequence) targeting Bst DNA polymerase via noncovalent binding has been selected using the systematic evolution of ligands by exponential enrichment (SELEX). The Bst DNA polymerase with the bound aptamer cannot perform strand displacement unless the temperature is raised to 50°C, thereby minimizing the unwanted isothermal preamplification usually occurring at room temperature, and mispriming is therefore prevented. Another attempt for limiting undesired preamplification and spurious results is by performing all sample preparation steps in ice before starting the reaction. By this simple tuning combined with the best DNA polymerase, the detections for *C. elegans*, *E. coli*, λ-phage specific genes, and Hela cell genomic DNA showed rapid (~10 min) and consistent isothermal amplification [51, 52].

2.1.4 Multiplex SDA reaction

The detection of more than one target from a single sample is usually required in medical diagnosis. Multiplexing is mainly achieved using spatial separation of targets, regional separation by targeting specific sites, or label-based techniques [53]. Though spatial and regional separation methods are highly employed for on-site multiplexed detection of various targets, they still suffer from expensive apparatus and complicated procedures [54, 55]. An alternative method is target-labeling approach, which uses different molecular recognition elements (dyes, enzymes, DNA probes, beads, aptamers, etc.) to identify different targets.

Primer design and optimization are essential for multiplex SDA. Singleplex SDA requires four primers to detect one target; therefore, duplexed detection would require eight primers, and so on. Thus, the number of primers increases rapidly with the number of targets. The large number of primers increases the complexity of the multiplex amplification system and therefore decreases the stability of the system. To solve this problem, Walker et al. developed a method called "adapter-mediated duplex SDA" for simultaneous detection of *Mycobacterium species* using fewer primers and without altering amplification yield [20]. In this method, a single pair of amplification primers and adapter sequences is used, where two target strands are amplified exponentially using dual primers. The first primer is attached to one end of the second target, while the second primer is appended to one end of the first target sequence. After amplification of the target strands by the primers, the adapter sequences start to bind to the amplified target sequences and begin extension and displacement, which results in a cascade of exponential amplification of the target sequences using the adapters rather than the primers. This method was also used for multiplexed SDA of three distinct DNA sequences of *Mycobacterium tuberculosis* and other mycobacteria [56]. Furthermore, multiplex SDA was used to amplify multiple SNPs simultaneously with molecular beacon probe-assisted fluorescent signal readout [57]. Most recently, several *BRCA* mutations were genotyped by combining SDA and mass spectrometry. Allele-specific regions were amplified and then ligated to adapters by DNA ligase, and the ligated products were SDA amplified with universal primers. The resulting fragments were analyzed and confirmed using mass spectrometry [58]. Though, this SDA method required complex equipment, it was able to detect hundreds of mutations.

2.1.5 Sample preparation

Isothermal amplification usually requires specimen isolation and culture, enzymatic treatment or genomic DNA (gDNA) extraction, and/or heat denaturation (in case of dsDNA) to obtain template DNA. Traditional sample preparation methods like genomic DNA extraction are time consuming and susceptible to contamination. Thus, crude cell lysate method is widely used, whereby cells are heat killed or enzymatically pretreated using proteinase K to expose DNA ready for amplification [59]. Cell cultures are usually heated at 92–95°C for 3–5 min and cooled to appropriate SDA temperature prior to the reaction. An up to date approach termed HUDSON (heating unextracted diagnostic samples to obliterate nucleases) combines the dual range of heating, that is, one temperature (37–50°C, 5–20 min) for nuclease inactivation, and another temperature (64–95°C, 5–20 min) for pathogen inactivation and genome exposure [60]. Though heat-assisted amplification is still frequently preferred owing to its simplicity, but it cannot differentiate nucleic acids from live and dead cells. As solution, Tong and colleagues used a set of restriction enzymes and modified nucleotides that could target different sites of target template and create a site of nicking and extension for SDA target DNA amplification [61]. However, these modified nucleotides and probes are costly, and the restriction enzymes exhibit random target digestion, which results in high background, low sensitivity, and specificity. Alternatively, heat treatment can also be abolished by using an improved SDA approach that initiates amplification at a DNA breaching site (Hoogsteen pairing), though its specificity to long templates is still of concern [3, 62].

To overcome contamination and detect live targets accurately, gDNA extraction free isothermal amplification methods have been adopted, which use extracellular compartment recognizing molecules such as aptamers. We reported ultrasensitive aptamer-based biosensors for the detection of live pathogens including *E. coli* and *S. enteritidis* [15, 24, 36]. In these methods, a dual aptamer system recognizing two extracellular membrane components are used. One bacterium-targeting aptamer is modified with biotin in order to react with streptavidin-coated magnetic beads during positive selection, while another bacterium-targeting aptamer is used as a template for SDA amplification. The bacteria-aptamer-magnetic bead complex is enriched, amplified, and applied to lateral flow strip for visual detection (**Figure 2**). This method sensitivity to pathogens is 10 *cfu* of live cells, therefore reduces false-positive results.

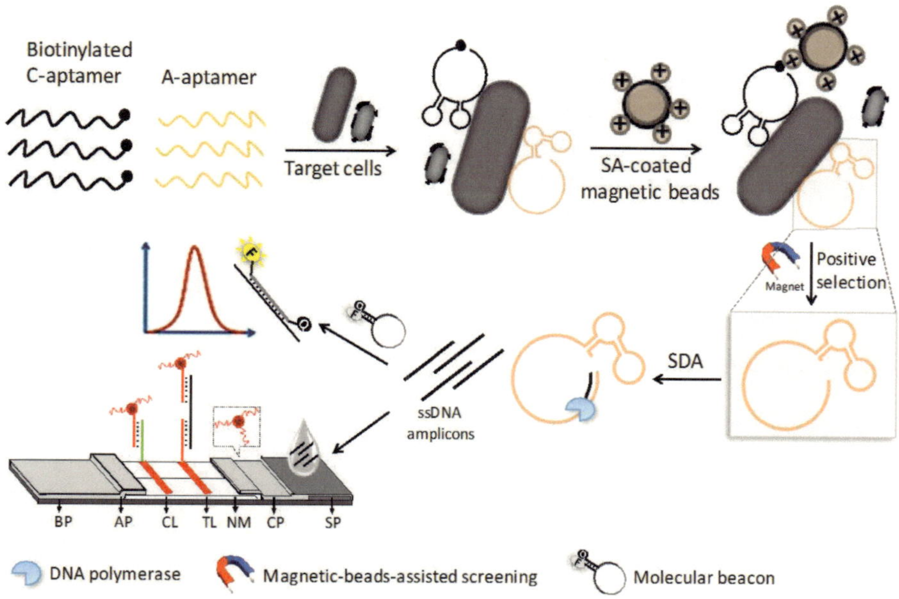

Figure 2. Conceptual illustration of SDA and aptamer-based nucleic acid biosensor. Two target-specific aptamers termed biotinylated capture aptamers (C-aptamer) and amplifying aptamers (A-aptamer) bind to target cells, for the enrichment of targeted cells and strand displacement amplification (SDA), respectively. After the binding reaction, streptavidin (SA)-coated magnetic beads are added to form cell-magnetic bead-aptamer complexes that are collected for SDA amplification. Finally, the single strand amplicons are loaded onto the lateral flow strip for visual readout or hybridized to fluorophore-probe after displacement of quencher-labeled probe for fluorescent detection.

3. SDA product analysis

Detection of amplified product is critical in isothermal amplification of nucleic acids, which includes quantification of the final amplification product and monitoring of the product during the process of amplification. Hereafter, we introduce a variety of methods for the detection of nucleic acids, which include intercalating fluorescent dyes, fluorescent probes, lateral flow biosensors, and CRISPR/Cas system.

3.1 Fluorescent dye-based analysis

Fluorescent gel staining dyes such as SYBR Green and ethidium bromide are commonly used for monitoring and quantitation of nucleic acids. SYBR Green I can intercalate into dsDNA, which emits light under UV-light. SYBR Green II is supersensitive to RNAs and ssDNA; however, it fluoresces in the presence of dsDNA or ssDNA [50]. Although SYBR Green is the most sensitive dyes employed to monitor nucleic acid amplification progress, high concentration of SYBR Green can inhibit SDA amplification [47]. Thus, other dyes such as Picogreen, Ribogreen, and Oligogreen have been developed. These versatile fluorescent dyes are specific, sensitive, and rapid for a broad spectrum of applications such as nucleic acid typing, amplification, and purification, Band-shift assays as well as DNA-damage assays. Interestingly, they are not interfered by free nucleotides and proteins. They are much more specific than

UV-based absorbance (A_{260}) and much easier to use than laborious radioisotope labeling and silver staining. They have been widely applied to quantitatively detect the early onset of diseases with window periods such as virus, oncogenes, etc. Furthermore, DNA dyes such as EMA (ethidium monoazide bromide azide) and PMA (propidium monoazide bromide azide) have been extensively used to distinguish nucleic acids of live and dead cells [63, 64]. These dyes can penetrate damaged cells and bind to DNA with little effect on live cells endowed from their intact cell membranes [65, 66]. However, their off-target binding and background result in spurious amplicon staining [47, 50] and are limited to single-strand conformation polymorphism (not at the level of single nucleotide polymorphism) [67].

3.2 Fluorescent probe-based analysis

To increase specificity, fluorescent oligo probes such as TaqMan probes and molecular beacons have been used to monitor and quantify nucleic acid amplification products [68–70]. A fluorescent probe consists of a fluorophore and a quencher covalently attached at 5′ and 3′ ends of a DNA probe sequence. There are two main types of fluorescent oligo probes, TaqMan probes and molecular beacons. In TaqMan probes, the fluorescent light of the fluorophore (e.g., FAM) is absorbed by the quencher (e.g., TAMRA) before amplification; therefore, no fluorescence can be detected. During amplification, the fluorescent probe hybridizes complementary to the target sequence, and the DNA polymerase degrades the probe via its 5′-3′ exonuclease activity. As a result, the fluorescent reporter and the quencher are separated, and the fluorescent reporter is then detected [71]. This technology has been widely used in real time PCR for medical diagnosis.

TaqMan probes depend on probe hybridization, polymerase extension, and cleavage of the probes. Molecular beacons, on the other hand, do not require polymerase extension and cleavage activity. Molecular beacons comprise modified stem ends with fluorescent and quencher molecules, a hairpin loop probe sequence (~20–25 bases) and complementary stem sequences (~4–6 base pairs). Before hybridization with the target sequence, the fluorophore on one end of the molecular beacon is quenched by the quencher on the other end of the beacon as the two ends are close together. When the probe hybridizes with the target nucleic acid sequence, the molecular beacon sequence becomes linear. As a result, the fluorophore and the quencher are separated, and the fluorescence is then detected. For example, the putative molecular beacon probes with fluorophore (5-(2′-aminoethyl)aminonaphthalene-1-sulfonic acid (EDANS)) and quencher (4-(4′-dimethylaminophenylazo) benzoic acid (DABCYL)) changes conformation and fluoresces spontaneously upon perfect complementarity with the target nucleic acid (**Figure 2**) [72]. This approach is best used to detect ssDNA products produced from SDA. It can also been multiplexed using multicolored molecular beacons for different targets [69].

Organic dyes such as rhodamine are conventionally used in fluorescent oligo probes. However, organic dyes have low quantum yield and are easily photo bleached. Other fluorophores such as quantum dots (QDs), silver nanoclusters, upconversion nanoparticles, and corresponding quenchers such as gold nanoparticles and carbon nanomaterials have been used to replace organic fluorophores and quenchers [73] for nuclei acid as well as protein detection [74, 75]. These nanomaterials have high quantum yield and photostability. In addition, they can be simultaneously excited using one wavelength during multiplex detection of various targets.

They are promising substitutes of organic dyes in the detection of nucleic acid detection using fluorescent oligo probes.

Tavares et al. reported an on-chip immobilization of QDs as energy donors in FRET and Cy3-labeled dsDNA target as a receiver for transduction of nucleic acid hybridization, which resulted in rapid quantitative determination of nucleic acid at the fmol level within 7 min after target introduction [76]. Silver nanoclusters possess much higher photostability and fluorescence than organic fluorophores and QDs, which have been used to detect influenza specific nucleic acids. Upon hybridization, these DNA-silver nanocluster probes fluoresce up to 500-fold when placed near G-rich nucleic acid targets and exhibited high signal to background ratio [77]. This finding was promising; however, it was elusive how fluorescence increased upon G-rich target detection. It is speculated that upon target binding guanines, G-quadruplex structures may be formed to yield reddish nanoclusters, or serve as electron donors since guanines have lowest oxidation potential compared with other nucleotides [78], or otherwise reduce oxidized nanoclusters and render them reddish [79, 80].

3.3 Lateral flow biosensor

Lateral flow biosensor is the most commonly used technology for the point of care testing [81–84]. A test strip consists of four parts: a sample pad, a conjugate pad, a nitrocellulose membrane, and an absorption pad. This method uses fiber chromatography material as a solid phase to allow capillary flow of sample solution, followed by the reaction between the analyte in the sample and the target recognition molecules fixed on the nitrocellulose membrane [9] (**Figure 2**). Color development can be obtained through enzymatic reaction, or visually detectable materials such as gold nanoparticles.

For the detection of nucleic acids, traditional lateral flow biosensor has been modified and termed nucleic acid lateral flow biosensor. In nucleic acid lateral flow biosensors, antibodies or antigens are replaced with probe DNAs that are fixed on the test zone and control zone to capture specific targets via nucleic acid hybridization. Based on SDA and aptamers, we developed a nucleic acid lateral flow biosensor to detect as low as 1 cfu/ml of pathogens, 1 ppm heavy metals, SNPs, and stem cells [15, 24] (**Figure 2**). This nucleic acid biosensor consists of (i) a specific capture probe, complementary to one part of the target nucleic acid and conjugated on gold nanoparticles, (ii) a target-hybridizing probe, immobilized on the nitrocellulose membrane test zone to capture amplified target sequence, and (iii) a specific nucleic acid probe on control zone that can hybridize with nanoparticle labeled probe. The hybridization on test line occurs at the presence of target, while in the absence of target sequence, the test zone does not show up. The appearance of the control zone shows the assay works properly. This method is fast, specific, sensitive, and cost effective. With different targeting aptamers and corresponding test zones on the test strip, multiplexing assay can be developed to detect multiple pathogens [84].

3.4 CRISPR-Cas-based analysis of nucleic acids

CRISPR-Cas is known to endow bacteria and archaea adaptive immunity against foreign nucleic acids using mobile genetic elements [85]. CRISPR-Cas proteins cleave invading DNA and generate spacer nucleotides known as protospacer. The protospacer integrates into genome near the protospacer adjacent motif (PAM) region required as memory for future interrogation and cleavage of same invader depending on spacer-phage similarity. For the targeting, CRISPR-Cas9 requires a gRNA (guide RNA) composed of *tracr*RNA (trans-activating) and crRNA, or a chimeric sgRNA (single guide RNA). The RNA-guided cleavage is mediated by RuvC (a member of RNase H family) and HNH catalytic domains at the site of gRNA-target sequence base-pairing. In this mechanism, Cas9-gRNA complex recognizes a G-rich PAM region of the target sequence followed by blunt end cleavage. However, some Cas enzymes such as Cas9 and Cas12a, purified from *Francisella tularensis novicida* and *Streptococcus pyogenes,* exhibit nonspecific RNA-independent DNA cleavage in the presence of $Mn2^{+}$ [86], suggesting the significant role of several mediators including Cas RuvC nuclease domain. On the basis of gRNAs, more literatures indicated that Cas12a, Cas13a, and Cas13b enzyme effectors require a mature crRNA for self-assembly and processing and ribonucleoprotein surveillance-dependent nuclease or DNA for interference activity [87, 88]. Moreover, the Cas12a, Cas13a, and Cas13b enzymes do not require a dual functional crRNA-TrancRNA as for Cas9 [89, 90].

Basically, CRISPR-Cas systems are categorized into three main types (type I, type II, and type III) and 12 subclasses based on the genetic and structural differences [91]. From these classes, Type II CRISPR-Cas is widely used for genome-editing applications. Currently, researchers have exploited the CRISPR-Cas system in diagnostics. Two CRISPR-Cas-based diagnostic systems termed DETECTR (DNA Endonuclease Targeted CRISPR *Trans* Reporter) and SHERLOCK (Shorthand for Specific High Sensitivity Reporter unLOCKing) have been developed as a new platform for real time detection of nucleic acid based on Type II Cas13a and Cas12a, respectively. These enzymes exhibit collateral cleavage of nucleic acid targets and nontarget single strands in vicinity. For instance, Cas13, an RNA-targeting CRISPR-associated type VI-A protein, cleaves an ssRNA at a non-G PFS (protospacer flanking site) of target sequence in a gRNA-independent manner via its endonuclease HPN domain [12]. On the contrary of Cas13a and distinct from Cas9, Cas12a (cpf1) is a CRISPR-Cas family enzyme that possess a unique RNA-guided DNase activity [88]. It targets at 5′ T-rich PAM region (TTTN) by cleaving ~18 nucleotides on the DNA strand opposite to the gRNA complementary strand by leaving 5 nucleotide staggered cuts on both 5′-ends of the target sequence [92]. Cas12a can collaterally cleave both targeted dsDNA and a nontarget ssDNA in vicinity. Through the integration of a fluorescently labeled ssDNA reporter, a detectable signal can be obtained after cleavage. However, the cleavage of reporter nucleic acids is motif dependent and requires 41–44 nucleotide crRNA to recognize a 5′ T-rich PAM of the target sequence, while Cas9 requires ~100 nucleotide gRNA at the 3′G-rich PAM target site. Nevertheless, Cas12a is unable to *trans*-cleave an ssRNA reporter and a targeted ssRNA sequence [11], suggesting that it exhibits only a DNA-activated DNase activity. In contrast, Cas13 enzymes (e.g., CcaCas13b and LwaCas13b) from some bacteria strains have shown a random enriched motif cleavage with U-dependent nucleotide preference, while some other Cas13 enzymes (e.g., PsmCas13b and AsCas12a) strongly preferred A-nucleotides and A-T dinucleotide across the motif, respectively [11]. Nevertheless, other CRISPR-Cas13a/b exhibited dinucleotide preference collateral cleavage activity. This activity can be enhanced with optimized target concentration, buffer, and crRNAs. Therefore, irrespective of the target

http://dx.doi.org/10.5772/intechopen.80687

efficiency of the CRISPR/Cas system, it is consent that a single-guided RNA-Cas enzyme complex recognition of target nucleic acid and reaction conditions is required to initiate cleavage of both target and a nearby nontarget (reporter sequence).

Various diagnostic applications necessitate detection of one or more targets, and therefore with tremendous propensity of both platforms, CRISPR-Cas enzymes can detect a single or multiple targets in complex liquid biopsy samples. Various samples suspected with Zika, dengue, and human papilloma viruses and bacteria as well as SNP and mutation discrimination have been developed. Their multiplex detection relies on reprogrammable crRNA tailing specific target sequence and enriched multiple motif fluorescent reporters. For example, Gootenberg et al. showed that isothermally amplified four different target nucleic acids could be detected simultaneously by LwaCas13a, PsmCas13b, CcaCas13b, and AsCas12a, with leveraged dinucleotide motifs harboring FAM, TEX, Cy5, and HEX quenched fluorescent reporters, respectively. After, the reporter is cleaved by Cas enzymes; the read-out can be achieved by high specific detection of four different quenched fluorescent reporters or using lateral flow biosensor analysis with specific antibodies against fluorescein-biotin reporters at conjugate pad and protein A as second antibody immobilized at the control line (**Figure 3**). Thus, these enzymes are intriguing for broad spectrum diagnostic applications (**Figure 3,** left). Moreover, the combination of isothermal amplification and CRISPR-Cas system for amplification and signal readout, respectively, revealed an amplified signal detection of 8zM in a 250 μl reaction volume. It should be noted that isothermal preamplification of target nucleic acids is crucial to achieve that robust sensitivity with Cas12 and Cas13 enzymes [13]. This approach could be adopted, however with the most minimized cost. More interestingly, it is simple, fast, specific, sensitive, and can be multiplexed. Thus, it is convenient in minimally instrumented fields for point-of-care detection of nucleic acids.

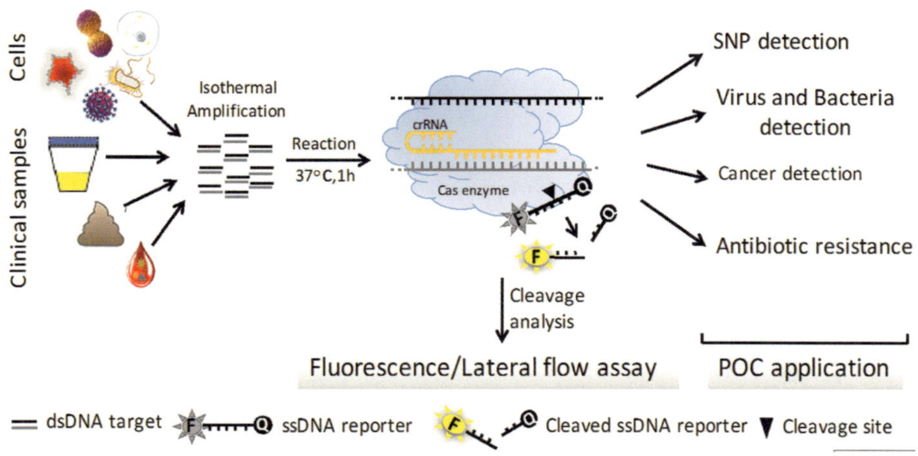

Figure 3. Workflow of nucleic acid detection with the CRISPR-Cas system. Nucleic acids are obtained from samples by proteinase K treatment or heat treatment. The nucleic acids are isothermally amplified using recombinase polymerase amplification at 37°C for 10 min. A one-pot reaction comprising amplicons, Cas protein, a designed crRNA for specific DNA/RNA target spotting, and reporters is prepared. To detect the presence of target nucleic acid, a fluorophore molecule (yellow star) and a quenching molecule (circle) are used. When Cas protein slices its nucleic acid target, and any ssDNA reporter nearby, the quenching molecule frees from the fluorophore, letting it fluoresce. The fluorescence can be detected directly or the reaction mixture can be applied to lateral flow assay.

4. Discussion, conclusion, and future perspectives

The development of new methodologies in nucleic acid amplification is of great importance in point of care diagnosis for research and public health. The SDA and its colleagues such as RPA, LAMP, etc. have proved reliable application for this purpose. Nevertheless, SDA has poorly achieved longer sequence amplification and a comparable amplification as for LAMP toward turbidity measurement, but under stringent conditions, possesses higher sensitivity, specificity, and cost-efficiency, and can be multiplexed and reprogrammed for various targets [58, 93–96]. But also, other isothermal amplification methods such as LAMP have hardly shown multiplexing capacity [97–99] and are solely dye dependent for colorimetric detection and quantification, which are target independent and nonspecific. Up to now, no perfect method can overcome all shortcomings. However, probe-based lateral flow assay in combination with SDA could provide robust multiplexing detection higher than their peer antibodies [84]. For example, our group [15, 24, 36] and other researchers [3, 100, 101] demonstrated that SDA can be used to amplify short target recognition sequences, for example, aptamers, after target binding and then integrated with lateral flow biosensors for analysis. Therefore, preheat denaturation of templates, background signals, and unspecificity encountered during the use of long nucleic acid templates or the presence of DNA contaminants are prevented [102, 103]. Furthermore, the lab-on chip approach, consisting of on-chip fixed multiple analytes, could eliminate partially primer-dimerization frequently observed during multiplexed isothermal amplification [104].

DNA fluorescent probes were widely applied for singlex and multiplex detection of isothermal amplified nucleic acid targets. Notwithstanding, comparing with fluorescent probe detection of nucleic acids and other PCR-based techniques, CRISPR-Cas-based analysis of isothermal amplified products is fast, sensitive, and specific, allowing its on-site implementation. This technique is reprogrammable for the ultrasensitive and specific detection of various targets and is amenable to multiplexing by using their targeting Cas proteins and fluorescent labels [11, 13, 60]. Nevertheless, further studies are still needed to overcome some drawbacks of this technology. For example, the cost of enzymes and anti-fluorophore reporters still needs to be reduced. Moreover, the operability needs to be improved because the usage of more enzymes in one reaction requires complicated optimization for one-pot concurrent catalysis. In the lateral flow assay, we propose the combination of CRISPR-Cas with DNA capture probe technique for the cleaved and noncleaved reporters' detection, in order to replace the immunoassay approaches which are prone to cross reactivity. Furthermore, the sensitivity of this emerging diagnosis depends solely on target (s) nucleic acid (s) amplification. Thus, alternatively, one can develop an intrinsic signal amplification of reporters' signal by either cationic and fluorescent conjugated polymers or direct inhibition of fluorescent loss using fluorophore encapsulation. For signal amplification, the CRISPR system might be promoted by using other fluorescent-intensity-based nanostructures (e.g., quantum dots and silver nanostructures) and up conversion nanomaterials alongside with robust quenchers such as gold nanoparticles [105] and carbon nanomaterials (graphene oxides and single-walled carbon nanotubes) [106]. Additionally, the use of G-quadruplex-mediated catalysis for colorimetric detection of isothermal amplified amplicons or cleaved-CRISPR reporters could eliminate the need of more enzymes and thus allow conveniently the one-pot reaction toward simplified, cost-effective, specific, and sensitive on-site detection of nucleic acids.

Acknowledgements

We acknoledge the High-Level Talent Start-Up Research Project of Foshan University (gg07034, gg07016), Wuhan Enterprise Technology Innovation Project (2018020402011228) and the project of the department of education of Guangdong Province (Young Creative Talents, Natural Science, No. 2017KQNCX217).

Conflict of interest

The authors declare no competing financial interest.

Author details

Lingwen Zeng[1,2]*, Omar Mukama[2,3], Xuewen Lu[2], Shilin Cao[1] and Donghai Lin[1]

*Address all correspondence to: zeng6@yahoo.com

1 School of Food Science and Engineering, Foshan University, Foshan, China

2 Key Laboratory of Regenerative Biology, South China Institute for Stem Cell Biology and Regenerative Medicine, Guangzhou Institutes of Biomedicine and Health, Chinese Academy of Sciences, Guangzhou, China

3 Department of Applied Biology, College of Science and Technology, University of Rwanda, Kigali, Rwanda

References

[1] Borst A et al. Clinical evaluation of a NASBA-based assay for detection of Candida spp. in blood and blood cultures. Clinical Laboratory. 2002;**48**(9-10):487-492

[2] Walker GT et al. Strand displacement amplification—an isothermal, in vitro DNA amplification technique. Nucleic Acids Research. 1992;**20**(7):1691-1696

[3] Toley BJ et al. Isothermal strand displacement amplification (iSDA): A rapid and sensitive method of nucleic acid amplification for point-of-care diagnosis. Analyst. 2015; **140**(22):7540-7549

[4] Zhang Z, Birkedal V, Gothelf KV. Enzyme-free colorimetric detection systems based on the DNA strand displacement competition reaction. New Journal of Physics. 2016; **18**(5):055002

[5] Giuffrida MC, Spoto G. Integration of isothermal amplification methods in microfluidic devices: Recent advances. Biosensors & Bioelectronics. 2017;**90**:174-186

[6] Mori Y, Notomi T. Loop-mediated isothermal amplification (LAMP): A rapid, accurate, and cost-effective diagnostic method for infectious diseases. Journal of Infection and Chemotherapy. 2009;**15**(2):62-69

[7] Ali MM et al. Rolling circle amplification: A versatile tool for chemical biology, materials science and medicine. Chemical Society Reviews. 2014;**43**(10):3324-3341

[8] Lobato IM, O'Sullivan CK. Recombinase polymerase amplification: Basics, applications and recent advances. TrAC Trends in Analytical Chemistry. 2018;**98**:19-35

[9] Vincent M, Xu Y, Kong H. Helicase-dependent isothermal DNA amplification. EMBO Reports. 2004;**5**(8):795-800

[10] Jeong Y-J, Park K, Kim D-E. Isothermal DNA amplification in vitro: The helicase-dependent amplification system. Cellular and Molecular Life Sciences. 2009;**66**(20):3325

[11] Chen JS et al. CRISPR-Cas12a target binding unleashes indiscriminate single-stranded DNase activity. Science. 2018;**360**(6387):436-439

[12] Abudayyeh OO et al. RNA targeting with CRISPR-Cas13. Nature. 2017;**550**(7675):280-284

[13] Gootenberg JS et al. Multiplexed and portable nucleic acid detection platform with Cas13, Cas12a, and Csm6. Science. 2018;**360**(6387):439-444

[14] Cosentino LA, Landers DV, Hillier SL. Detection of *Chlamydia trachomatis* and *Neisseria gonorrhoeae* by strand displacement amplification and relevance of the amplification control for use with vaginal swab specimens. Journal of Clinical Microbiology. 2003;**41**(8):3592-3596

[15] Fang Z et al. Lateral flow biosensor for DNA extraction-free detection of salmonella based on aptamer mediated strand displacement amplification. Biosensors and Bioelectronics. 2014;**56**:192-197

[16] Shi C et al. Highly sensitive chemiluminescent point mutation detection by circular strand-displacement amplification reaction. Biosensors and Bioelectronics. 2011;**26**(12): 4697-4701

[17] Wang L et al. Reverse strand-displacement amplification strategy for rapid detection of p53 gene. Talanta. 2018;**187**:365-369

[18] Shi C et al. Exponential strand-displacement amplification for detection of microRNAs. Analytical Chemistry. 2014;**86**(1):336-339

[19] Maragh S et al. Multiple strand displacement amplification of mitochondrial DNA from clinical samples. BMC Medical Genetics. 2008;**9**(1):7

[20] Walker GT et al. Multiplex strand displacement amplification (SDA) and detection of DNA sequences from *Mycobacterium tuberculosis* and other mycobacteria. Nucleic Acids Research. 1994;**22**(13):2670-2677

[21] Li Y et al. Fluorometric determination of Simian virus 40 based on strand displacement amplification and triplex DNA using a molecular beacon probe with a guanine-rich fragment of the stem region. Microchimica Acta. 2017;**184**(2):557-562

[22] Zhang P et al. A label-free ultrasensitive fluorescence detection of viable *Salmonella enteritidis* using enzyme-induced cascade two-stage toehold strand-displacement-driven assembly of G-quadruplex DNA. Biosensors and Bioelectronics. 2016;**80**:538-542

[23] Wu W et al. Aligner-mediated cleavage of nucleic acids and its application to isothermal exponential amplification. Chemical Science. 2018;**9**(11):3050-3055

[24] Wu W et al. A sensitive lateral flow biosensor for Escherichia coli O157:H7 detection based on aptamer mediated strand displacement amplification. Analytica Chimica Acta. 2015; **861**:62-68

[25] Walker GT, Linn CP, Nadeau JG. DNA detection by strand displacement amplification and fluorescence polarization with signal enhancement using a DNA binding protein. Nucleic Acids Research. 1996;**24**(2):348-353

[26] Lu W et al. Self-primed isothermal amplification for genomic DNA detection of human papillomavirus. Biosensors & Bioelectronics. 2017;**90**:258-263

[27] Mehrpouyan M et al. A rapid and sensitive method for non-isotopic quantitation of HIV-1 RNA using thermophilic SDA and flow cytometry. Molecular and Cellular Probes. 1997;**11**(5):337-347

[28] Motley ST et al. Improved multiple displacement amplification (iMDA) and ultraclean reagents. BMC Genomics. 2014;**15**:443

[29] Lee CY et al. Rapid and label-free strategy for the sensitive detection of Hg2+ based on target-triggered exponential strand displacement amplification. RSC Advances. 2017;**7**(74): 47143-47147

[30] Yin J et al. Engineering a universal and label-free evaluation method for mycotoxins detection based on strand displacement amplification and G-quadruplex signal amplification. Sensors and Actuators B: Chemical. 2018;**256**:573-579

[31] Li J et al. A fluorescence biosensor for VEGF detection based on DNA assembly structure switching and isothermal amplification. Biosensors and Bioelectronics. 2017;**89**:964-969

[32] Lee CY, Park KS, Park HG. A simple, sensitive, and label-free assay for alkaline phosphatase activity based on target-promoted exponential strand displacement amplification. Sensors and Actuators B: Chemical. 2018;**262**:1001-1005

[33] Wu D et al. A label-free colorimetric isothermal cascade amplification for the detection of disease-related nucleic acids based on double-hairpin molecular beacon. Analytica Chimica Acta. 2017;**957**:55-62

[34] Xu X et al. An integrated and restructive probe mediated strand displacement amplification strategy for sensitive and specific DNA methyltransferase activity detection. Sensors and Actuators B: Chemical. 2018;**266**:124-130

[35] Dong H et al. A biofunctional molecular beacon for detecting single base mutations in cancer cells. Molecular Therapy - Nucleic Acids. 2016;**5**:e302

[36] Wu W et al. Strand displacement amplification for ultrasensitive detection of human pluripotent stem cells. Analytica Chimica Acta. 2015;**881**:124-130

[37] He J-L et al. Fluorescence aptameric sensor for strand displacement amplification detection of cocaine. Analytical Chemistry. 2010;**82**(4):1358-1364

[38] Wang M et al. Signal-on electrochemiluminescence biosensor for microRNA-319a detection based on two-stage isothermal strand-displacement polymerase reaction. Biosensors and Bioelectronics. 2018;**107**:34-39

[39] Ge B et al. Identification of *Escherichia coli* O157:H7 and other enterohemorrhagic serotypes by EHEC-hly A targeting, strand displacement amplification, and fluorescence polarization. Molecular and Cellular Probes. 2002;**16**(2):85-92

[40] Phillips EA et al. Strand displacement probes combined with isothermal nucleic acid amplification for instrument-free detection from complex samples. Analytical Chemistry. 2018;**40**(11):6580-6586

[41] Qu X et al. Strand displacement amplification reaction on quantum dot-encoded silica bead for visual detection of multiplex microRNAs. Analytical Chemistry. 2018;**90**(5): 3482-3489

[42] Bellamy SRW et al. Cleavage of individual DNA strands by the different subunits of the heterodimeric restriction endonuclease BbvCI. Journal of Molecular Biology. 2005; **348**(3):641-653

[43] Heiter DF, Lunnen KD, Wilson GG. Site-specific DNA-nicking mutants of the heterodimeric restriction endonuclease R.BbvCI. Journal of Molecular Biology. 2005;**348**(3):631-640

[44] Zhu Z et al. Engineering strand-specific DNA nicking enzymes from the type IIS restriction endonucleases BsaI, BsmBI, and BsmAI. Journal of Molecular Biology. 2004; **337**(3):573-583

[45] Zhang P et al. Engineering BspQI nicking enzymes and application of N.BspQI in DNA labeling and production of single-strand DNA. Protein Expression and Purification. 2010;**69**(2):226-234

[46] Xu SY, Zhu Z, Chan SH, Xu Y. Recombinant DNA nicking endonuclease and uses thereof. United States Pantent Application Publication, US 2008/0268507 A1. 2008. p. 37

[47] Joneja A, Huang X. Linear nicking endonuclease-mediated strand-displacement DNA amplification. Analytical Biochemistry. 2011;**414**(1):58-69

[48] Chan S-h et al. Cloning of CviPII nicking and modification system from chlorella virus NYs-1 and application of Nt.CviPII in random DNA amplification. Nucleic Acids Research. 2004;**32**(21):6187-6199

[49] Xu Y, Lunnen KD, Kong H. Engineering a nicking endonuclease N.AlwI by domain swapping. Proceedings of the National Academy of Sciences of the United States of America. 2001;**98**(23):12990-12995

[50] Tan E et al. Specific versus nonspecific isothermal DNA amplification through thermophilic polymerase and nicking enzyme activities. Biochemistry. 2008;**47**(38):9987-9999

[51] Little MC et al. Strand displacement amplification and homogeneous real-time detection incorporated in a second-generation DNA probe system, BDProbeTecET. Clinical Chemistry. 1999;**45**(6 pt 1):777-784

[52] Kaneko H et al. Tolerance of loop-mediated isothermal amplification to a culture medium and biological substances. Journal of Biochemical and Biophysical Methods. 2007;**70**(3):499-501

[53] Dincer C et al. Multiplexed point-of-care testing—xPOCT. Trends in Biotechnology. 2017;**35**(8):728-742

[54] Araz MK, Tentori AM, Herr AE. Microfluidic multiplexing in bioanalyses. Journal of Laboratory Automation. 2013;**18**(5):350-366

[55] Gordon J, Michel G. Discerning trends in multiplex immunoassay technology with potential for resource-limited settings. Clinical Chemistry. 2012;**58**(4):690-698

[56] Badak FZ et al. Confirmation of the presence of *Mycobacterium tuberculosis* and other mycobacteria in mycobacterial growth indicator tubes (MGIT) by multiplex strand displacement amplification. Journal of Clinical Microbiology. 1997;**35**(5):1239-1243

[57] Huang Y et al. Multiple sample amplification and genotyping integrated on a single electronic microarray. Electrophoresis. 2004;**25**(18-19):3106-3116

[58] Park JH et al. A mass spectrometry-based multiplex SNP genotyping by utilizing allele-specific ligation and strand displacement amplification. Biosensors and Bioelectronics. 2017;**91**:122-127

[59] Zhong J, Zhao X. Isothermal amplification technologies for the detection of foodborne pathogens. Food Analytical Methods. 2018;**11**(6):1543-1560

[60] Myhrvold C et al. Field deployable viral diagnostics using CRISPR-Cas13. Science. 2018; **360**(6387):444-448

[61] Tong Y. 3 - Isothermal amplification of specific sequences. In: Schaudies RP, editor. Biological Identification. Woodhead Publishing; 2014. pp. 69-92

[62] Frank-Kamenetskii MD, Prakash S. Fluctuations in the DNA double helix: A critical review. Physics of Life Reviews. 2014;**11**(2):153-170

[63] Lv X-C et al. Development of propidium monoazide combined with real-time quantitative PCR (PMA-qPCR) assays to quantify viable dominant microorganisms responsible for the traditional brewing of Hong Qu glutinous rice wine. Food Control. 2016;**66**:69-78

[64] Elizaquivel P, Aznar R, Sanchez G. Recent developments in the use of viability dyes and quantitative PCR in the food microbiology field. Journal of Applied Microbiology. 2014;**116**(1):1-13

[65] Andorrà I et al. Determination of viable wine yeast using DNA binding dyes and quantitative PCR. International Journal of Food Microbiology. 2010;**144**(2):257-262

[66] Delgado-Viscogliosi P, Solignac L, Delattre JM. Viability PCR, a culture-independent method for rapid and selective quantification of viable *Legionella pneumophila* cells in environmental water samples. Applied and Environmental Microbiology. 2009;**75**(11): 3502-3512

[67] Rodriguez A et al. Design of primers and probes for quantitative real-time PCR methods. Methods in Molecular Biology. 2015;**1275**:31-56

[68] Tyagi S, Bratu DP, Kramer FR. Multicolor molecular beacons for allele discrimination. Nature Biotechnology. 1998;**16**:49

[69] Tyagi S, Kramer FR. Molecular beacons: Probes that fluoresce upon hybridization. Nature Biotechnology. 1996;**14**(3):303

[70] Lie YS, Petropoulos CJ. Advances in quantitative PCR technology: 5′ nuclease assays. Current Opinion in Biotechnology. 1998;**9**(1):43-48

[71] Kong D-M et al. Duplex probes: A new approach for the detection of specific nucleic acids in homogenous assays. Analytica Chimica Acta. 2003;**491**(2):135-143

[72] Matsuo T. In situ visualization of messenger RNA for basic fibroblast growth factor in living cells. Biochimica et Biophysica Acta (BBA) - General Subjects. 1998;**1379**(2):178-184

[73] Chan WC. Quantum dot bioconjugates for ultrasensitive nonisotopic detection. Science. 1998;**281**(5385):2016-2018

[74] Ding Y et al. Gold nanoparticles for nucleic acid delivery. Molecular Therapy. 2014;**22**(6):1075-1083

[75] Su X et al. Nucleic acid fluorescent probes for biological sensing. Applied Spectroscopy. 2012;**66**(11):1249-1261

[76] Tavares AJ et al. On-chip transduction of nucleic acid hybridization using spatial profiles of immobilized quantum dots and fluorescence resonance energy transfer. Analytical Chemistry. 2012;**84**(1):312-319

[77] Yeh H-C et al. A DNA–silver nanocluster probe that fluoresces upon hybridization. Nano Letters. 2010;**10**(8):3106-3110

[78] Rusalov MV, Druzhinin SI, Uzhinov BM. Intramolecular fluorescence quenching of crowned 7-aminocoumarins as potential fluorescent chemosensors. Journal of Fluorescence. 2004;**14**(2):193-202

[79] Sauer M et al. Dynamics of the electron transfer reaction between an oxazine dye and DNA oligonucleotides monitored on the single-molecule level. Chemical Physics Letters. 1998;**284**(3):153-163

[80] Torimura M et al. Fluorescence-quenching phenomenon by photoinduced electron transfer between a fluorescent dye and a nucleotide base. Analytical Sciences. 2001;**17**(1): 155-160

[81] Du X-J et al. Rapid detection of *Staphylococcus aureus* via recombinase polymerase amplification combined with lateral flow strip. Food Analytical Methods. 2018;**11**(8):2296-2306

[82] Han J et al. Nanozyme-based lateral flow assay for the sensitive detection of *Escherichia coli* O157:H7 in milk. Journal of Dairy Science. 2018;**101**(7):5770-5779

[83] Zhao F et al. Rapid and sensitive detection of *Pseudomonas aeruginosa* using multiple cross displacement amplification and gold nanoparticle-based lateral flow biosensor visualization. FEMS Microbiology Letters. 2018;**365**(14)

[84] Zheng W et al. Lateral flow test for visual detection of multiple MicroRNAs. Sensors and Actuators B: Chemical. 2018;**365**:320-326

[85] Barrangou R et al. CRISPR provides acquired resistance against viruses in prokaryotes. Science. 2007;**315**(5819):1709-1712

[86] Sundaresan R et al. RNA-independent DNA cleavage activities of Cas9 and Cas12a. Cell Reports. 2017;**21**(13):3728-3739

[87] Swarts DC, van der Oost J, Jinek M. Structural basis for guide RNA processing and seed-dependent DNA targeting by CRISPR-Cas12a. Molecular Cell. 2017;**66**(2):221-233.e4

[88] Gao P et al. Type V CRISPR-Cas Cpf1 endonuclease employs a unique mechanism for crRNA-mediated target DNA recognition. Cell Research. 2016;**26**(8):901-913

[89] Brouns SJ et al. Small CRISPR RNAs guide antiviral defense in prokaryotes. Science. 2008;**321**(5891):960-964

[90] Deltcheva E et al. CRISPR RNA maturation by trans-encoded small RNA and host factor RNase III. Nature. 2011;**471**(7340):602-607

[91] Shmakov S et al. Diversity and evolution of class 2 CRISPR–Cas systems. Nature Reviews Microbiology. 2017;**15**:169

[92] Chen JS, Doudna JA. The chemistry of Cas9 and its CRISPR colleagues. Nature Reviews Chemistry. 2017;**1**(10):0078

[93] Wu W et al. Aligner-mediated cleavage-triggered exponential amplification for sensitive detection of nucleic acids. Talanta. 2018;**185**:141-145

[94] Mayboroda O, Katakis I, O'Sullivan CK. Multiplexed isothermal nucleic acid amplification. Analytical Biochemistry. 2018;**545**:20-30

[95] Wang Y et al. Multiplex, rapid, and sensitive isothermal detection of nucleic-acid sequence by endonuclease restriction-mediated real-time multiple cross displacement amplification. Frontiers in Microbiology. 2016;**7**(753)

[96] Nyan DC et al. Rapid detection of hepatitis B virus in blood plasma by a specific and sensitive loop-mediated isothermal amplification assay. Clinical Infectious Diseases. 2014;**59**(1):16-23

[97] Notomi T et al. Loop-mediated isothermal amplification of DNA. Nucleic Acids Research. 2000;**28**(12):e63-e63

[98] Fukuma A et al. Rapid detection of Lassa virus by reverse transcription-loop-mediated isothermal amplification. Microbiology and Immunology. 2011;**55**(1):44-50

[99] Blomstrom AL et al. A one-step reverse transcriptase loop-mediated isothermal amplification assay for simple and rapid detection of swine vesicular disease virus. Journal of Virological Methods. 2008;**147**(1):188-193

[100] He Y et al. Visual detection of gene mutations based on isothermal strand-displacement polymerase reaction and lateral flow strip. Biosensors and Bioelectronics. 2012;**31**(1):310-315

[101] Deng X et al. Applying strand displacement amplification to quantum dots-based fluorescent lateral flow assay strips for HIV-DNA detection. Biosensors and Bioelectronics. 2018;**105**:211-217

[102] Cogswell FB et al. Host DNA can interfere with detection of *Borrelia burgdorferi* in skin biopsy specimens by PCR. Journal of Clinical Microbiology. 1996;**34**(4):980-982

[103] Sachse S et al. Truncated human cytidylate-phosphate-deoxyguanylate-binding protein for improved nucleic acid amplification technique-based detection of bacterial species in human samples. Journal of Clinical Microbiology. 2009;**47**(4):1050-1057

[104] Kunze A et al. On-chip isothermal nucleic acid amplification on flow-based chemiluminescence microarray analysis platform for the detection of viruses and bacteria. Analytical Chemistry. 2016;**88**(1):898-905

[105] Saidi A, Mirzaei M, Zeinali S. Using antibody coated gold nanoparticles as fluorescence quenchers for simultaneous determination of aflatoxins (B1, B2) by soft modeling method. Chemometrics and Intelligent Laboratory Systems. 2013;**127**:29-34

[106] Leng X et al. Circular exponential amplification of photoinduced electron transfer using hairpin probes, G-quadruplex DNAzyme and silver nanocluster-labeled DNA for ultrasensitive fluorometric determination of pathogenic bacteria. Microchimica Acta. 2018;**168**(3)

Chapter 6

MultiSite Gateway Technology Is Useful for Donor DNA Plasmid Construction in CRISPR/Cas9-Mediated Knock-In System

Takeshi Yasuda and Katsushi Tajima

Additional information is available at the end of the chapter

http://dx.doi.org/10.5772/intechopen.80775

Abstract

The clustered regulatory interspaced short palindromic repeats (CRISPR)/Cas9 method is a powerful tool for genome editing, by introducing a DNA double-strand break (DSB) at the specific site. The gene knock-out can be achieved by the deletion or insertion at the CRISPR/Cas9-mediated DSB site by error-prone nonhomologous end joining repair in targeted cells. However, the gene knock-in is still difficult as compared to the knock-out, because of the low efficiency of homology directed repair with donor DNA in cells. Therefore, to efficiently select the knock-in cells, we developed a complicated donor DNA plasmid containing an antibiotic-resistance gene, in addition to the knock-in sequence and the two homology arms. MultiSite Gateway technology is a useful tool for constructing this complicated plasmid. We describe the MultiSite Gateway technology and provide an overview of the DSB repair pathways to clarify the knock-out and knock-in methods by the CRISPR/Cas9 system.

Keywords: knock-in, homology directed repair (HDR), MultiSite Gateway, donor DNA plasmid, CRISPR/Cas9, DSB repair

1. Introduction

Genome editing has been an important technique to investigate gene function in biology since before the development of the clustered regulatory interspaced short palindromic repeats (CRISPR)/Cas9 system. In microorganisms such as *Escherichia coli (E. coli)* and yeast, gene disruption can be achieved by simply introducing a donor DNA into the cells without inducing a DSB in the targeted gene [1–3]. With regards to gene disruption in vertebrate cells, chicken B lymphocyte line DT 40 cells have been widely used because of their high efficiency of homologous DNA recombination [4–6]. Similar to *E. coli* and yeast cells, gene disruption in DT 40 cells can also be achieved by introducing a DNA vector for gene targeting into the cells. In contrast, gene disruption by this method in human cells is difficult, because of the inefficient homologous recombination in the cells. Therefore, gene knockdown by RNA interference (RNAi) has usually been used in human cells, in order to examine the functions of human genes [7]. However, the targeted protein cannot be completely eliminated from the cells by RNAi. Therefore, an efficient method for targeted gene disruption in human cells has been keenly desired.

The CRISPR/Cas9 method is an innovative genome editing technology. The history of this technology originated from the finding of unusual, functionally unknown repeated sequences in *E. coli* [8, 9]. In the repeated sequences, highly homologous repeats are separated by nonrepetitive nucleotides as spacers. Repeated sequences, composed of repeats and spacers, were also found in numerous genomes of other bacteria and archaea [10] and were named CRISPR [11]. In addition, well-conserved genes were identified adjacent to the CRISPR loci and were named CRISPR-associated (Cas) genes [11]. Some of the Cas protein families were found to share sequence homology with proteins involved in DNA metabolism, such as helicases and exonucleases [11], and the purified Cas proteins exhibited endonuclease activity [12–14]. Sequences identical to the CRISPR spacers were found among bacterial mobile genetic elements, such as plasmids and phages, suggesting that the CRISPR spacers in the bacterial genome are derived from DNA fragments of the invading foreign genetic elements [15, 16]. In bacteria, CRISPR/Cas serves as a defense system against the invasion of mobile genetic elements [17]. The molecular mechanism of the defense system was elucidated by biochemical experiments [13, 14, 18, 19]. Cas proteins bind to RNA transcribed from the CRISPR spacer sequence and cleave the precursor CRISPR RNA (pre-crRNA) [18]. Cas proteins exist in the complex with the cleaved mature crRNA [18] and cleave invading foreign genetic elements mediated by the crRNA guide, containing the complementary sequence with the targeted genetic elements [13, 14, 19]. Among the Cas family proteins, a single Cas9 protein complexed with a crRNA can introduce a specific DSB at the desired site in the target DNA [13, 14]. Therefore, the CRISPR/Cas9 system is being applied for genome engineering [20, 21]. The biology and technology of the CRISPR/Cas system are described in detail in excellent reviews [22–27].

A variety of CRISPR/Cas9-mediated genome editing tools is now commercially available. A gene knock-out can be accomplished simply by using the CRISPR/Cas9 tool. However, for a gene knock-in or replacement, a donor DNA must also be prepared individually. Here, we describe the usefulness of the MultiSite Gateway technology [28, 29] for the construction of the donor DNA plasmid.

2. DSB repair pathways involved in genome editing

The CRISPR/Cas9-mediated gene knock-out or knock-in is based on the mechanisms of DSB repair. To better understand the genome editing by the CRISPR/Cas9 method, we first provide an overview of the DSB repair mechanisms.

DSBs are repaired by multiple mechanisms [30] (**Figure 1**). One of the major DSB repair mechanisms is nonhomologous end joining (NHEJ). NHEJ is the simplest method for DSB repair,

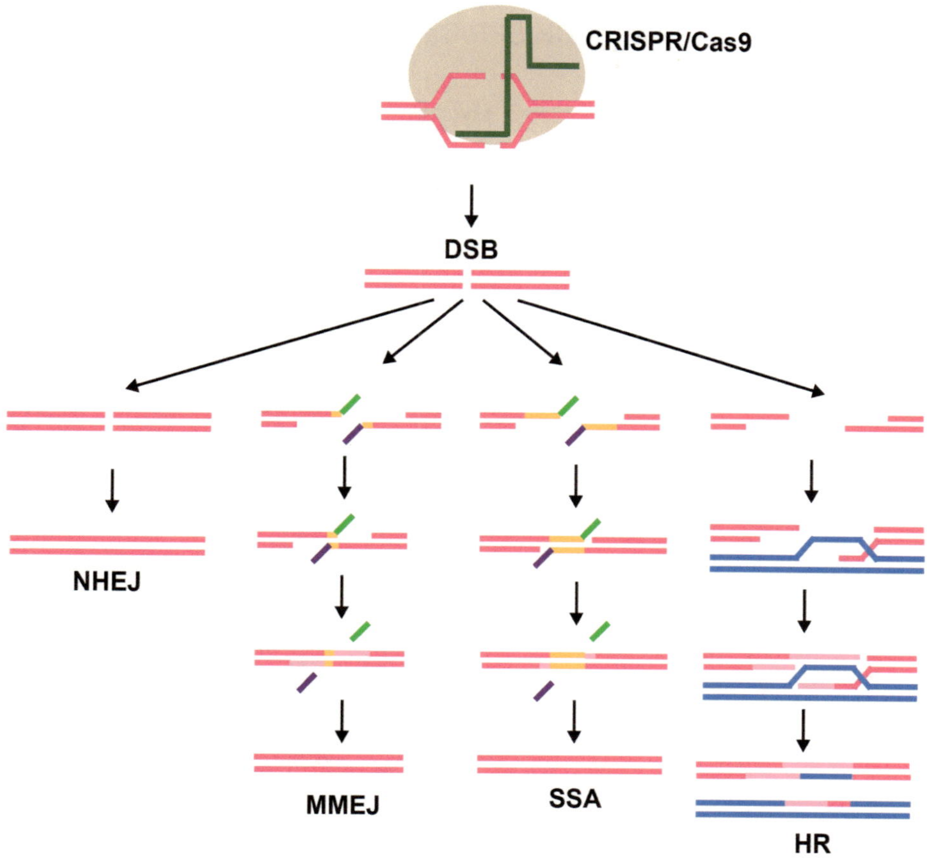

Figure 1. Multiple DSB repair pathways. The targeted DSB induced by CRISPR/Cas9 is repaired by NHEJ, MMEJ, SSA, or HR.

in which the broken ends of the DNA are rejoined, and is a rapid and predominant DSB repair pathway in mammalian cells [31]. The DSB is accurately repaired to its normal state when the broken ends are protected during repair. However, if the broken ends are digested before rejoining, the DNA information at or around the DSB site is lost. Thus, NHEJ is an error-prone DSB repair pathway [32]. CRISPR/Cas9-mediated gene knock-out technology utilizes this mutagenic aspect of NHEJ, and thus requires only DSB induction in the targeted gene. Most of the DSBs are repaired accurately by NHEJ [33]. However, if the DSB site is repaired accurately, then the target DNA site seems to be attacked repeatedly by CRISPR/Cas9, until the site is broken and thus insensitive to the hybridization with the crRNA (**Figure 2**). This apparently enhances the knock-out efficiency by CRISPR/Cas9.

The second major DSB repair pathway is homologous DNA recombination (HR) [34, 35] (**Figure 1**). In HR, DSBs are repaired by DNA strand exchange with the undamaged homologous DNA strand. In *E. coli* or yeast, HR is the predominant mechanism for DSB repair. In the first step of HR, the DSB ends are resected by a nuclease to generate 3′ single-strand (ss) DNA overhangs. Then, the ssDNA overhangs invade and anneal with the undamaged homologous DNA strand. New DNA is synthesized from the 3′ end of the invaded DNA as a primer, according to the sequence information of the undamaged DNA template, thereby

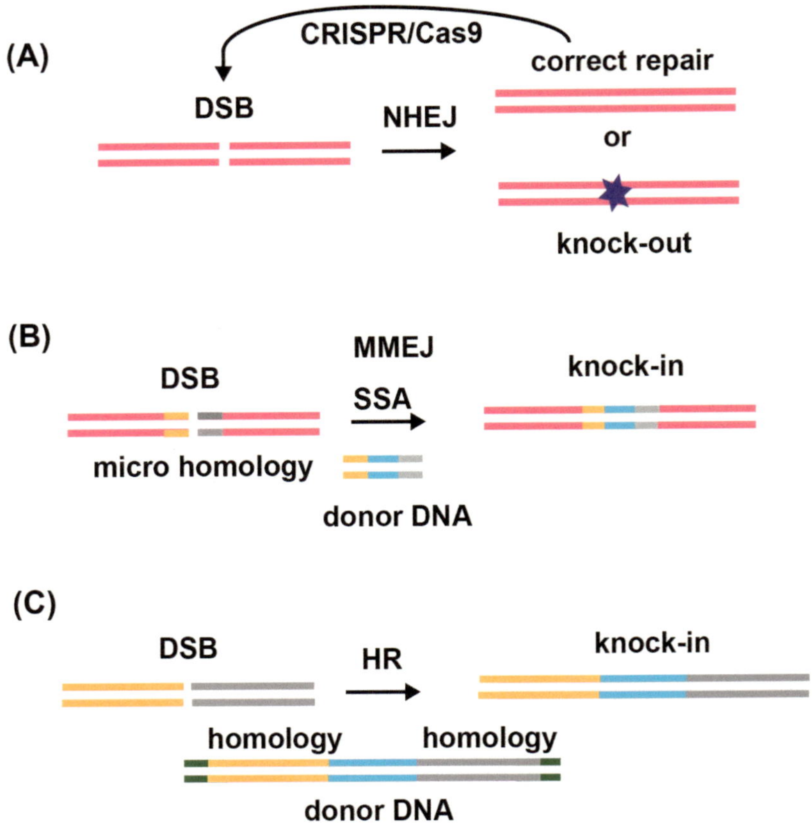

Figure 2. Gene knock-in or knock-out by DSB repair pathways. (A) Targeted gene disruption induced by NHEJ. (B) Targeted short DNA fragment insertion mediated by MMEJ or SSA. (C) Targeted long DNA fragment insertion mediated by HR.

restoring the lost sequence information at the damaged sites. The branch point in the crossed DNA strands moves during the repair process. Finally, the crossed DNA strands are resolved by cutting and rejoining. Thus, the DNA information can be restored by HR repair even if the broken DNA ends are digested, such as by nucleases. Therefore, HR is a more precise DSB repair mechanism, as compared to NHEJ. If the homologous DNA strand is available in the donor DNA, then the donor DNA is integrated into the damaged site by HR (**Figure 2**). Thus, HR is an important mechanism for a gene knock-in.

DSBs are also repaired by other mechanisms, including microhomology-mediated end joining (MMEJ) and single-strand annealing (SSA) (**Figure 1**). Although MMEJ and SSA are mechanistically similar, they are distinct pathways with different repair proteins. Both MMEJ and SSA use relatively short internal homologous sequences flanking both sides of the DNA break. The length of the homologous sequence required for MMEJ is shorter than that for SSA. The first step of MMEJ or SSA is the resection of the DSB site, and thereby the homologous dsDNA region becomes ssDNA. In the next step, the ssDNA regions with the homologous sequence are annealed, and the 3′ flaps of the nonhomologous region are removed. Finally, the gapped

DNA regions are filled by DNA synthesis, and the resulting nicks are rejoined [36–39]. Both repair pathways induce a DNA deletion at the damaged site, and therefore could contribute to the CRISPR-Cas9-mediated gene knock-out in the absence of a DNA donor [40, 41]. However, when the donor DNA is provided, the repair pathways can be used for gene knock-in [42–44] (**Figure 2**).

3. Donor DNA plasmid for homology directed gene knock-in

The knock-in of a relatively short gene fragment (up to ~1.5 kb) can be achieved by MMEJ or SSA with a linearized donor DNA fragment containing short (about 20–60 bp) homologous DNA regions, called homology arms [42, 43, 45–47]. The knock-in efficiency decreases as the size of the insert DNA increases [48]. In the case of the insertion of a long DNA fragment (more than 1.5 kb), the knock-in efficiency increased as the length of the homology arms increased, up to about 1500 bp [48]. Thus, long homology arms (more than 500 bp) are usually used for the knock-in of such a long DNA fragment [45, 49–52]. In this case, the knock-in is mediated by HR. The knock-in efficiency by HR is low [53], and accordingly, a selectable marker is introduced into the donor DNA plasmid for screening the knock-in clones in some cases [49–52]. Therefore, the selectable donor DNA plasmid for the HR-mediated gene knock-in contains left and right arms, the inserted gene of interest, and a selectable marker gene with promoter and transcription terminator regions. An example of a donor DNA plasmid is shown in **Figure 3** [52]. In our donor DNA plasmid, the left and right arms contain the promoter and transcription terminator regions of the inserted gene of interest, respectively. However, the native transcription terminator region is separated from the gene of interest by the neighboring selectable

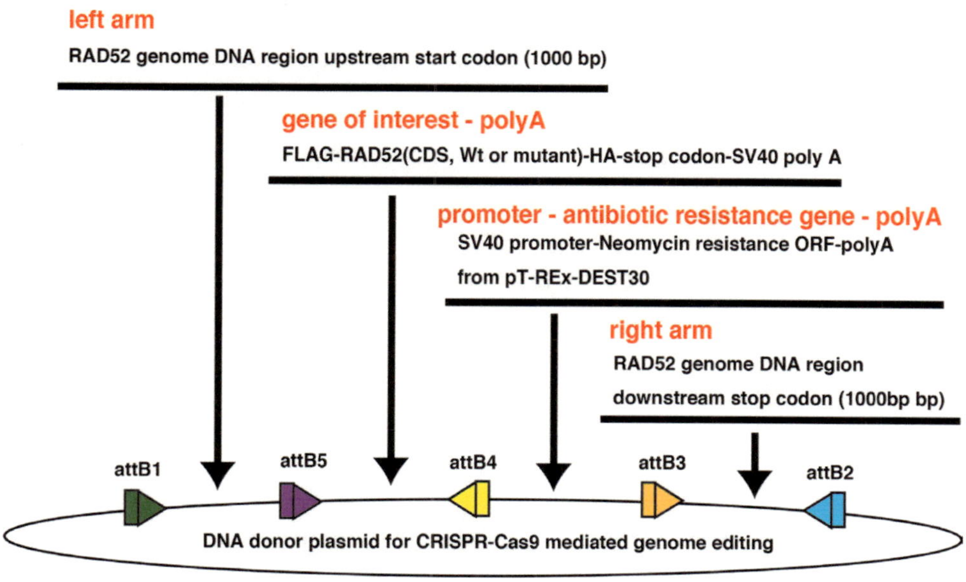

Figure 3. A donor DNA plasmid for HR-mediated gene knock-in.

marker gene. Therefore, the SV40 transcription terminator sequence is also placed just downstream of the gene of interest. Thus, the structure of the donor DNA plasmid is complicated, as it contains multiple inserted DNA regions. It is difficult to construct such a complicated plasmid by using classical restriction enzyme-mediated cloning methods. In some cases, the donor DNA plasmids were constructed by a site-specific recombinational cloning method named In-Fusion technology [54], provided by Clontech [42, 55].

4. Gateway technology for DNA cloning

Gateway technology is another site-specific recombinational cloning method [54, 56] (**Figure 4**). This technology is based on the site-specific recombination system of *E. coli* bacteriophage λ [57]. Bacteriophage λ integrates into the *E. coli* chromosome by site-specific recombination between the attachment (*att*) sites on the *b*acterial chromosome (attB) and the *att* sites on the *p*hage chromosome (attP), to generate left (attL) and right (attR) att sites. This recombination

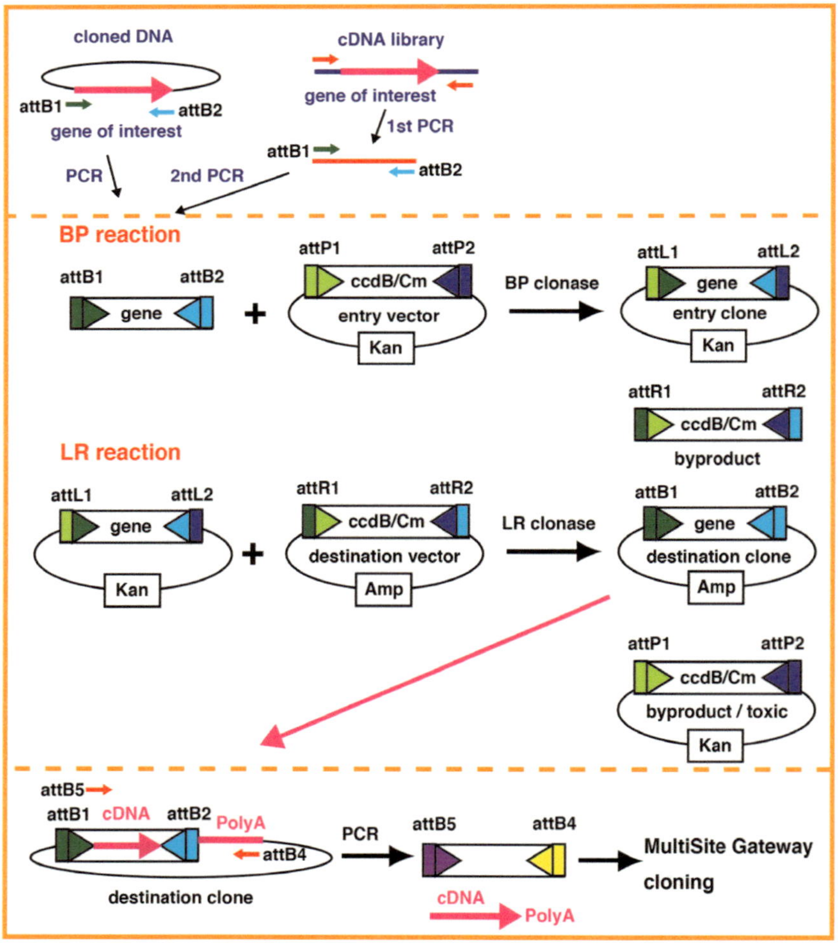

Figure 4. Standard Gateway method for single-fragment cloning. The DNA fragment of a gene of interest is amplified by PCR with a cloned DNA or cDNA library as the PCR template. The destination clone containing a polyadenylation (polyA) tail region downstream from the cDNA can be used as a PCR template for the next MultiSite Gateway cloning. Abbreviations: Kan, kanamycin resistance gene; Amp, ampicillin resistance gene; Cm, chloramphenicol resistance gene.

reaction is mediated by the integrase (Int) enzyme of bacteriophage λ and the integration host factor (IHF) of *E. coli.* The excision reaction requires another host factor, excisionase (Xis), in addition to Int and IHF. The Gateway technology has developed mutant att sites (such as attB1, attB2, attP1, and attP2) [56]. The attB1 site specifically recombines with the attP1 site, but not attP2, to generate the attL1 and attR1 sites. Similarly, the attB2 site specifically recombines with the attP2 site to generate the attL2 and attR2 sites.

In the first step of the Gateway cloning, the DNA fragment for cloning is amplified by PCR with primer sets containing attB1 or attB2 sequences at the 5′ ends (**Figure 4**). Gateway cloning vectors (pDONR) contain attP1 and attP2 sites for cloning. Therefore, the PCR product containing the attB1 or attB2 sites at both ends can be specifically inserted in between the attP1 and attP2 sites of the pDONR vector by site-specific recombination, to generate the entry clone of the Gateway system. A protein mixture (BP clonase) containing Int and IHF is used for this *in vitro* site-specific recombination reaction (BP reaction). In the pDONR vector, the *ccdB* gene from F factor of *E. coli* is located between the attP1 and attP2 sites. The CcdB protein is a toxin for *E. coli* cells that lack the antitoxin, the CcdA protein, which is also produced from F factor of *E. coli* [58–61]. Therefore, *E. coli* cells without F factor or the *ccdA* gene cannot grow, due to the production of the CcdB protein from the pDONR vector. For example, *E. coli* DH5α cells lack F factor and the *ccdA* gene. Therefore, the cell growth of the DH5α strain is inhibited in the presence of the pDONR vector. The Gateway cloning method applies this cell killing mechanism mediated by the *ccdB* gene for efficient DNA cloning. If the PCR product is successfully cloned between the attP1 and attP2 sites of the pDONR vector, then the *ccdB* gene is removed from the vector by the site-specific recombination. Therefore, when the *in vitro* site-specific reaction mixture is transformed into DH5α cells, only the cells containing the generated entry clone can grow. Thus, all of the transformed colonies contain the successfully cloned plasmid DNA. This is an excellent point of the Gateway cloning method. In the constructed entry clone, the cloned gene is present between the generated attL1 and attL2 sites.

The Gateway cloning system provides destination vectors for numerous purposes, such as for expressing the cloned gene in a variety of organisms. Each destination vector contains attR sites for cloning on both sides of the *ccdB* gene (**Figure 4**). The cloned gene in the entry clone can be transferred to destination vectors by an *in vitro* site-specific recombination reaction (LR reaction) between the attL and attR sites with a protein mixture (LR clonase) containing Int, IHF, and Xis, to generate the destination clone. As a result of the reaction, the *ccdB* gene of the destination vector is replaced with the gene of interest and is transferred to the pDONR vector as a by-product. Therefore, when the LR reaction mixture is transformed into DH5α cells, the growth of the cells containing the by-product plasmid is inhibited by the expression of the toxic *ccdB* gene. The antibiotic resistance gene of the destination vector is different from that of the pDONR vector. Therefore, only the desired destination clone is selected in the presence of the appropriate antibiotics. Thus, once the DNA fragment of interest is cloned into the pDONR vector, the DNA fragment can be transferred to a variety of destination vectors quite easily.

5. MultiSite Gateway technology for donor DNA plasmid construction

The original Gateway cloning system was further improved for cloning multiple DNA fragments into a single vector [28, 62]. The improved cloning method is called MultiSite Gateway

[29, 63] (**Figure 5**). In the MultiSite Gateway cloning method, numerous attB, attP, attL, and attR variant sites were developed. Each attB site is specifically recombined with the corresponding attP site by the BP reaction, to generate the corresponding attL and attR sites. Similarly, each attL

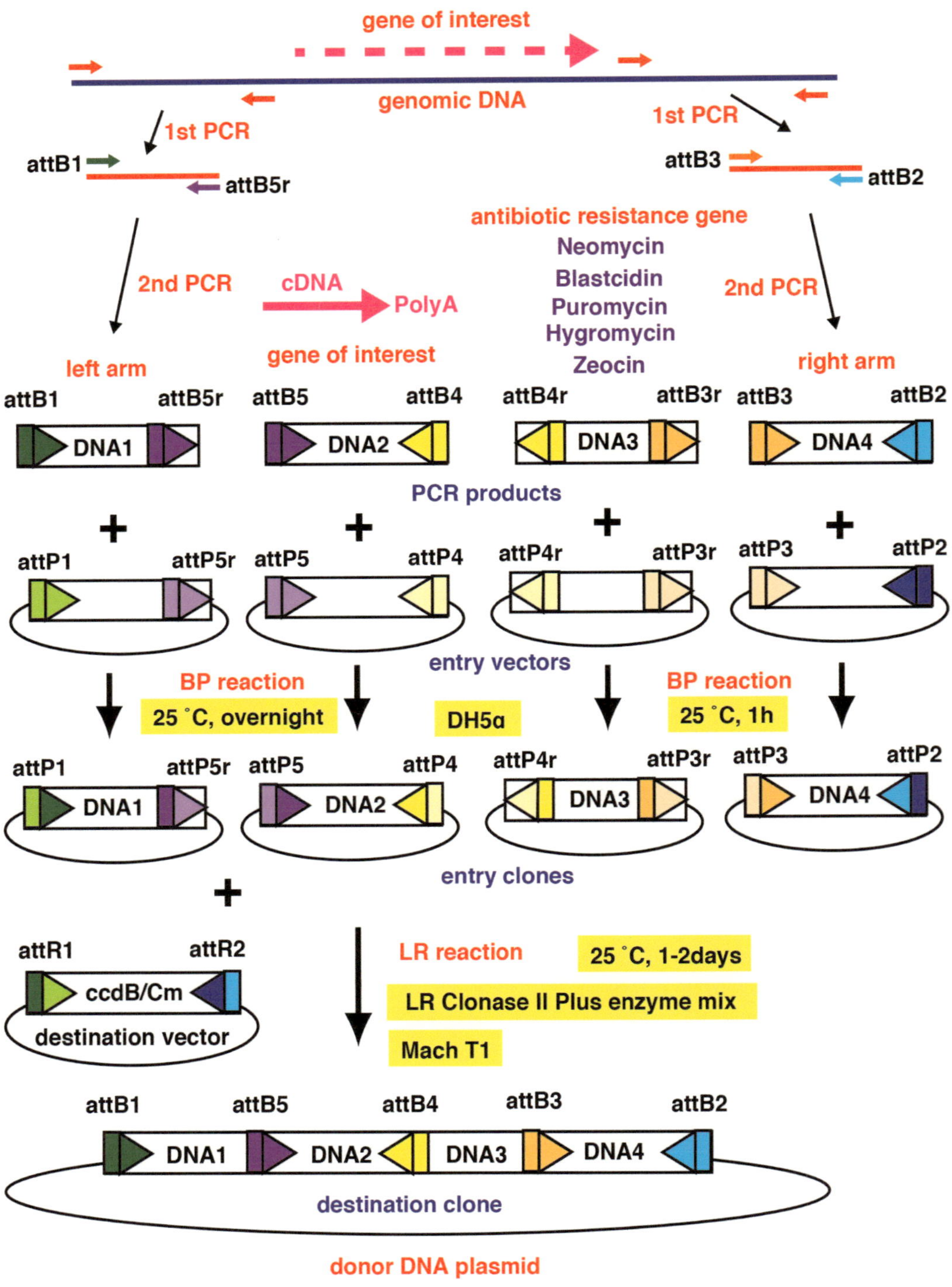

Figure 5. Cloning four-fragments by the MultiSite Gateway method. The strategy for the construction of the donor DNA plasmid is shown.

site is specifically recombined with the corresponding attR site by the LR reaction. At present, up to four DNA fragments can be cloned into a single vector. The 4-fragment MultiSite Gateway cloning technology is suitable for the construction of a donor DNA plasmid for CRISPR/Cas9 and HR-mediated gene knock-in (**Figure 5**). In the first step of the 4-fragment cloning, each PCR-amplified DNA fragment is cloned into the corresponding pDONR vectors. As shown in **Figure 5**, the orientation of the att site sequence is important. The attB3r, attB4r, and attB5r sequences are reversely oriented relative to the attB3, attB4, and attB5 sequences, respectively. In the second cloning step, the four entry clones are mixed with an appropriate destination vector and are subjected to the LR reaction. Thus, the four DNA fragments are simultaneously assembled and inserted into a single destination vector, in the desired order and orientation. The outline of our example is described below [52].

We used a CRISPR/Cas9-mediated gene knock-in, in order to express the wild type or mutant gene of interest (human RAD52 gene in our case) with its own native promoter in the genome and to examine the cellular effects of the mutant protein expressed at the endogenous level. The 1000 bp genomic DNA region upstream from the start codon of the gene of interest was amplified by PCR with primer sets containing attB1 or attB5r sequences at the 5′ ends and was cloned between the corresponding attP1 and attP5r sites of the first pDONR vector. The 1000 bp genomic DNA region downstream from the stop codon of the gene was cloned between the attP3 and attP2 sites of the fourth pDONR vector (**Figures 3** and **5**). The cDNA of the gene (wild type or mutant) was first cloned via standard Gateway cloning into a destination vector (pT-Rex-DEST30), for gene expression with the CMV promoter of the vector (**Figure 4**). In the destination clone, the SV40 polyadenylation region required for transcriptional termination is present downstream from the stop codon of the cloned gene. We amplified the DNA region encoding the cDNA of the gene and the SV40 polyadenylation region by PCR, using the destination clone as the PCR template. The PCR product was cloned between the attP5 and attP4 sites of the second pDONR vector (**Figure 5**). The DNA region containing the SV40 promoter, neomycin resistance gene, and polyadenylation region was amplified by PCR with pT-Rex-DEST30 as the PCR template and was cloned between the attP4r and attP3r sites of the third pDONR vector (**Figure 5**). The DNA fragments in each of the entry clones were verified by DNA sequencing. Then, the LR reaction was performed with the confirmed four types of entry clones and the destination vector (a simple vector, pDEST14, in our case). Thus, the complicated donor DNA plasmids could be constructed relatively easily, by using the MultiSite Gateway technology.

6. Advantages of MultiSite Gateway technology for donor DNA plasmid construction

MultiSite Gateway technology is suitable for the construction of a complicated donor DNA plasmid, for several reasons. In this method, all parts of the complicated donor DNA are first cloned into entry vectors, before their assembly. The cloned parts are easily verified by DNA sequencing. The verified entry clones can be used as parts for constructing other donor DNAs. For example, the entry clone containing the required part for expressing the neomycin resistance gene can be reused for constructing donor DNA plasmids targeting the other genes. For generating knock-in cells, other antibiotic (such as blasticidin, puromycin, hygromycin, and zeocin) resistance genes are sometimes required as the selection markers. In this case, if the

DNA fragments required for expressing the other antibiotic resistance genes are cloned into the entry vector, we can substitute the neomycin resistance gene of the donor DNA plasmid in **Figure 3** with the other antibiotic genes very easily (**Figure 5**). One of the purposes of generating knock-in cells is to elucidate the function and regulation of the gene product of interest, by expressing the mutants of the gene related to genetic diseases or altered protein modification sites. By using the MultiSite Gateway cloning method, the donor DNA plasmids containing a variety of mutant genes can be easily constructed by simply substituting only the entry clones containing the mutant genes of interest (**Figure 5**). For these reasons, MultiSite Gateway cloning is a convenient and useful method for constructing the complicated donor DNA plasmids.

7. Strategies and improvements for generating knock-in cells

To replace the whole endogenous gene with the donor gene, the targeted gene was cleaved around both the start and stop codons by the CRISPR/Cas9 method [52]. To avoid the cleavage of the donor vector, a specific cleavage sequence that does not exist within the donor DNA must be selected in the endogenous gene. Therefore, the targeted sequence for CRISPR/Cas9-mediated cleavage was designed within introns around both the start and stop codons of the gene. In our case, the cDNA of the donor gene contains FLAG and HA tag sequences at the amino (N)- and carboxyl (C)-terminal ends, respectively. Therefore, the DNA sequences around the start and stop codons are different and allow discrimination between the endogenous gene and the donor gene. By selecting the sequence containing the start or stop codon as the CRISPR/Cas9-targeted region, the endogenous gene can be cleaved selectively. For CRISPR/Cas9-mediated cleavage, a 5′-NGG-3′ sequence named the proto-spacer adjacent motif (PAM) is required on the 3′ end of the target sequence. In our case, PAM sequences were found in the vicinities of the start and stop codons of the target gene. Therefore, we could design the CRISPR RNAs to specifically guide Cas9 to the vicinity of the start or stop codon of the targeted endogenous gene. We used the commercially available GeneArt CRISPR Nuclease Vector from Life Technologies for the production of the CRISPR RNA and the Cas9 protein in cells. To generate the knock-in cells, the donor DNA plasmid was transfected into the cells with the two plasmids expressing the CRISPR RNAs targeting the vicinities of the start codon and the stop codon of the targeted gene. The transfected cells were initially cultured in the absence of selectable antibiotics for a few days and subsequently cultured in the presence of appropriate concentrations of the antibiotics for the selection of the knock-in cells. Most of the cells died after the selection. However, the antibiotic-resistant cells were observed after a long cultivation in the same culture dish. The antibiotic-resistant clones were isolated, the genomic DNA from each clone was purified, and the desired knock-in cells were subsequently verified by PCR and sequencing analyses. Thus, we obtained the desired knock-in cells by our method. However, we think that there is still room for improvements of our method.

In our method, we used circular plasmid DNA as the donor DNA (**Figure 3**). However, the knock-in efficiency is reportedly enhanced when the circular DNA is linearized [53]. Therefore, our strategy might be improved by using linearized donor DNA. According to the report, the knock-in efficiency of the donor DNA fragment is decreased when nonhomologous terminal DNA regions are present adjacent to the two homology arms [53]. The inhibitory effect of the nonhomologous DNA regions is increased in accordance with the length. Therefore, the most suitable donor DNA is a linearized DNA fragment containing homology arms at both terminal ends, without nonhomologous regions at the ends. When restriction enzyme sites are introduced at the terminal ends of the homology arms of our donor DNA plasmid, this linearized donor DNA can be produced by restriction enzyme cleavage. This modification of our strategy will improve the knock-in efficiency.

The DSB repair pathway choice is an important consideration to improve the knock-in efficiency. Among the several DSB repair pathways, the HR pathway choice is enhanced when the NHEJ pathway does not work [64]. Therefore, in order to increase the knock-in efficiency by HR, the inhibition of the NHEJ pathway was attempted in CRISPR/Cas9-mediated genome editing [65–68]. A chemical compound, SCR7, inhibits DNA ligase IV, which is an essential protein for NHEJ [69]. The CRISPR/Cas9-mediated homology-directed genome editing was enhanced by treating the cells with SCR7 [65, 66, 68]. In addition, a high throughput chemical screen identified small molecules that modulate CRISPR/Cas9-mediated genome editing [70]. The HR-mediated knock-in efficiency was improved by two chemical compounds, L755507 and BrefeldinA, which are a β3-adrenergic receptor agonist and an inhibitor of protein transport from the ER to the Golgi apparatus, respectively [70]. In contrast, the HR-mediated knock-in efficiency was decreased by the chemical compounds azidothymidine (AZT) and Trifluridine (TFT), which are anti-HIV and anti-herpes virus drugs, respectively [70]. In contrast to their effects on the HR-mediated knock-in, L755507 inhibits the NHEJ-mediated knock-out, whereas AZT enhanced it [70]. Therefore, in addition to their known activities, these chemical compounds could modulate the DSB repair pathway choice. The effectiveness of L755507 for the HR-mediated knock-in was also demonstrated in another study [68]. Therefore, the knock-in strategy could be further improved in combination with the usage of these chemical compounds.

8. Experimental procedure for donor DNA plasmid construction by MultiSite Gateway technology

Here, we describe our protocol for the donor DNA plasmid construction by the MultiSite Gateway technology.

8.1. PCR amplification of arm DNA fragments (1000 bp)

8.1.1. The first-round PCR

Primers (forward and reverse): arm DNA-specific oligonucleotides (35 mer)

Primer stocks (50 or 100 μM) are diluted to 10 μM prior to use.

Template: human genomic DNA, purified with a Blood & Cell Culture DNA Mini Kit (QIAGEN).

Template stock is diluted to 50 ng/μl prior to use.

PCR amplification is performed with PrimeSTAR GXL DNA Polymerase kit (Takara).

5X PrimeSTAR GXL buffer: 10 μl

dNTP Mixture (2.5 mM each): 4 μl

Forward primer (10 μM): 1 μl

Reverse primer (10 μM): 1 μl

Template (50 ng/μl): 1 μl

Sterile distilled water: 32 μl

PrimeSTAR GXL DNA Polymerase: 1 μl

PCR conditions

Initial step: 3 s at 98°C (denaturation)

25 cycles:

10 s at 98°C (denaturation)

15 s at 55°C (annealing)

1–2 min/kb at 68°C (extension)

Hold: 4°C (storage)

The PCR reaction mixture is purified with a QIAquick PCR Purification Kit (QIAGEN) to remove the PCR primers.

8.1.2. The second-round PCR

Forward primer for the left arm:

5′-GGGG-attB1 (ACAAGTTTGTACAAAAAAGCAGGCT)-(NN)-(template-specific sequence)-3′

Reverse primer for the left arm:

5′-GGGG-attB5r (ACAACTTTTGTATACAAAGTTG)T-(template-specific sequence)-3′

Forward primer for the right arm:

5′-GGGG-attB3 (ACAACTTTGTATAATAAAGTTG)-(NN)-(template-specific sequence)-3′

Reverse primer for the right arm:

5′-GGGG-attB2 (ACCACTTTGTACAAGAAAGCTGGGT)A-(template-specific sequence)-3′

The first-round primer sequences are used as each template-specific sequence.

If AA, AG, or GA is present 5′ of the template-specific sequence, then NN (except for AA, AG, or GA) is added in order to avoid the generation of a stop codon, as described in the MultiSite Gateway User Manual.

5X PrimeSTAR GXL buffer: 10 μl

dNTP Mixture (2.5 mM each): 4 μl

Forward primer (100 μM): 0.5 μl

Reverse primer (100 μM): 0.5 μl

Template (5 ng/μl): 2 μl

Sterile distilled water: 32 μl

PrimeSTAR GXL DNA Polymerase: 1 μl

PCR conditions

Initial step: 3 s at 98°C (denaturation)

10 cycles:

10 s at 98°C (denaturation)

1 min/kb at 68°C (annealing/extension)

Hold: 4°C (storage)

8.2. PCR amplification of the gene of interest (cDNA of the gene and polyadenylation region) or the antibiotic resistance gene (promoter, antibiotic resistance gene, and polyadenylation region)

Template: plasmid DNA

Forward primer for the gene of interest:

5′-GGGG-attB5 (ACAACTTTGTATACAAAAGTTG)-(NN)-Kozak sequence and start codon (ACCATG)-template-specific sequence)-3′

Reverse primer for the gene of interest:

5′-GGGG-attB4 (ACAACTTTGTATAGAAAAGTTGGGT)G-(template-specific sequence)-3′

Forward primer for the antibiotic resistance gene:

5′-GGGG-attB4r (ACAACTTTTCTATACAAAGTTG)-(NN)-(template-specific sequence)-3′

Reverse primer for the antibiotic resistance gene:

5′-GGGG-attB3r (ACAACTTTATTATACAAAGTTG)T-(template-specific sequence)-3′

If AA, AG, or GA is present 5′ of the template-specific sequence, then NN is added as above-mentioned.

5X PrimeSTAR GXL buffer: 10 µl

dNTP Mixture (2.5 mM each): 4 µl

Forward primer (100 µM): 0.5 µl

Reverse primer (100 µM): 0.5 µl

Template: 10 ng

PrimeSTAR GXL DNA Polymerase: 1 µl

Sterile distilled water: to final reaction volume of 50 µl

PCR conditions

Initial step: 3 s at 98°C (denaturation)

30–35 cycles:

10 s at 98°C (denaturation)

min/kb at 68°C (annealing/extension)

Hold: 4°C (storage)

If the template plasmid DNA contains a kanamycin resistance gene, which also exists in the pDONR entry vector, then the PCR reaction mixture is treated with the *Dpn*I enzyme to digest the template DNA.

The PCR products are purified by phenol/chloroform extraction and ethanol precipitation and are resuspended in TE buffer (10–50 µl).

8.3. BP reaction

pDONR entry vector (150 ng/µl; Invitrogen): 0.25 µl

BP Clonase II enzyme mix (Invitrogen): 0.5 µl

PCR product: 1–1.75 µl (10–100 ng)

TE buffer: to final reaction volume of 2.5 µl

Incubate at 25°C for 60 min (for attB4r/attB3r and attB3/attB2 fragments) or overnight (for attB1/attB5r and attB5/attB4 fragments).

(Note: the cloning efficiencies of the attB1/attB5r and attB5/attB4 fragments were low. A longer incubation time in the BP reaction improved the cloning efficiency.)

Add 0.25 μl Proteinase K solution (20 mg/ml; Invitrogen) to the reaction mixture. Incubate at 37°C for 10 min.

Transform the reaction mixture into DH5α competent cells by the heat-shock method. Spread the transformed cells on an LB agar plate containing 20 μg/ml of kanamycin and incubate it at 37°C overnight. The plasmids are purified from each colony on the LB agar plate and are verified by DNA sequencing.

8.4. MultiSite Gateway LR reaction

Destination vector (20 fmol/μl; Invitrogen): 0.5 μl

attB1/attB5r entry clone (10 fmol/μl): 0.5 μl

attB5/attB4 entry clone (10 fmol/μl): 0.5 μl

attB4r/attB3r entry clone (10 fmol/μl): 0.5 μl

attB3/attB2 entry clone (10 fmol/μl): 0.5 μl

TE buffer: 1.5 μl

LR Clonase II Plus enzyme mix (Invitrogen): 1 μl

(Note: LR Clonase enzyme and LR Clonase II enzyme mix, which are used for standard single fragment cloning, cannot be used for cloning multiple fragments.)

Incubate at 25°C for 1–2 days.

Add 0.5 μl Proteinase K solution (20 mg/ml; Invitrogen) to the reaction mixture. Incubate at 37°C for 10 min.

Transform the reaction mixture into Mach T1 competent cells (Invitrogen) by the heat-shock method. Spread the transformed cells on LB agar plates containing appropriate antibiotics and incubate them at 37°C overnight. The plasmid DNA is purified from the colonies on the LB agar plates and used as the donor DNA after verification.

(Notes: Mach T1 competent cells were more suitable for cloning multiple fragments than DH5α competent cells.)

9. Conclusion

The CRISPR/Cas9 technology has opened a new window to investigate gene functions by targeted knock-ins. By replacing the endogenous gene with the mutant gene, the cellular effects of the mutant can be examined under the most suitable native conditions of the gene expressed from the native promoter. The native expression level of the gene is also important for investigating the intracellular localization and behavior of the gene product, because over-expression of the gene by a nonnative promoter sometimes induces artifactual effects on the intracellular localization of the protein. The CRISPR/Cas9-mediated knock-in of specific tag sequences into the endogenous gene allows the investigation of the intracellular localization of the protein at the native expression level, by monitoring the introduced tag sequences. The construction of a complicated donor DNA is required for gene knock-in mediated by HR. This is a bottleneck point for the CRISPR/Cas9-mediated targeted knock-in technology. Standard Gateway cloning is a popular method for constructing ordinary expression plasmids and is therefore more commonly used as compared to MultiSite Gateway cloning. However, MultiSite Gateway cloning is a quite useful method, especially for constructing the complicated donor DNA plasmid. Therefore, this technology will contribute to the spread of CRISPR/Cas9-mediated targeted knock-in methods.

Acknowledgements

This work was supported by Grants-in Aid for Scientific Research from Japan Society for the Promotion of Science. This work was also supported by the general fund of NIRS, QST.

Conflict of interest

The authors declare no conflict of interest associated with this manuscript.

Author details

Takeshi Yasuda* and Katsushi Tajima

*Address all correspondence to: yasuda.takeshi@qst.go.jp

National Institute of Radiological Sciences (NIRS), National Institutes for Quantum and Radiation Sciences and Technology (QST), Chiba, Japan

References

[1] Ohmori H, Saito M, Yasuda T, Nagata T, Fujii T, Wachi M, et al. The *pcsA* gene is identical to *dinD* in *Escherichia coli*. Journal of Bacteriology. 1995;**177**:156-165

[2] Yasuda T, Morimatsu K, Horii T, Nagata T, Ohmori H. Inhibition of *Escherichia coli* RecA coprotease activities by DinI. The EMBO Journal. 1998;**17**:3207-3216. DOI: 10.1093/emboj/17.11.3207

[3] Brachmann CB, Davies A, Cost GJ, Caputo E, Li J, Hieter P, et al. Designer deletion strains derived from *Saccharomyces cerevisiae* S288C: A useful set of strains and plasmids for PCR-mediated gene disruption and other applications. Yeast. 1998;**14**:115-132. DOI: 10.1002/(SICI)1097-0061(19980130)14:2<115::AID-YEA204>3.0.CO;2-2

[4] Sonoda E, Sasaki MS, Buerstedde JM, Bezzubova O, Shinohara A, Ogawa H, et al. Rad51-deficient vertebrate cells accumulate chromosomal breaks prior to cell death. The EMBO Journal. 1998;**17**:598-608. DOI: 10.1093/emboj/17.2.598

[5] Winding P, Berchtold MW. The chicken B cell line DT40: A novel tool for gene disruption experiments. Journal of Immunological Methods. 2001;**249**:1-16

[6] Yamazoe M, Sonoda E, Hochegger H, Takeda S. Reverse genetic studies of the DNA damage response in the chicken B lymphocyte line DT40. DNA Repair. 2004;**3**:1175-1185. DOI: 10.1016/j.dnarep.2004.03.039

[7] Elbashir SM, Harborth J, Lendeckel W, Yalcin A, Weber K, Tuschl T. Duplexes of 21-nucleotide RNAs mediate RNA interference in cultured mammalian cells. Nature. 2001;**411**: 494-498. DOI: 10.1038/35078107

[8] Ishino Y, Shinagawa H, Makino K, Amemura M, Nakata A. Nucleotide sequence of the iap gene, responsible for alkaline phosphatase isozyme conversion in *Escherichia coli*, and identification of the gene product. Journal of Bacteriology. 1987;**169**:5429-5433

[9] Nakata A, Amemura M, Makino K. Unusual nucleotide arrangement with repeated sequences in the *Escherichia coli* K-12 chromosome. Journal of Bacteriology. 1989;**171**: 3553-3556

[10] Mojica FJ, Diez-Villasenor C, Soria E, Juez G. Biological significance of a family of regularly spaced repeats in the genomes of Archaea, Bacteria and mitochondria. Molecular Microbiology. 2000;**36**:244-246

[11] Jansen R, Embden JD, Gaastra W, Schouls LM. Identification of genes that are associated with DNA repeats in prokaryotes. Molecular Microbiology. 2002;**43**:1565-1575

[12] Beloglazova N, Brown G, Zimmerman MD, Proudfoot M, Makarova KS, Kudritska M, et al. A novel family of sequence-specific endoribonucleases associated with the clustered regularly interspaced short palindromic repeats. The Journal of Biological Chemistry. 2008;**283**:20361-20371. DOI: 10.1074/jbc.M803225200

[13] Jinek M, Chylinski K, Fonfara I, Hauer M, Doudna JA, Charpentier E. A programmable dual-RNA-guided DNA endonuclease in adaptive bacterial immunity. Science. 2012;**337**:816-821. DOI: 10.1126/science.1225829

[14] Gasiunas G, Barrangou R, Horvath P, Siksnys V. Cas9-crRNA ribonucleoprotein complex mediates specific DNA cleavage for adaptive immunity in bacteria. Proceedings of the National Academy of Sciences of the United States of America. 2012;**109**:E2579-E2586. DOI: 10.1073/pnas.1208507109

[15] Mojica FJ, Diez-Villasenor C, Garcia-Martinez J, Soria E. Intervening sequences of regularly spaced prokaryotic repeats derive from foreign genetic elements. Journal of Molecular Evolution. 2005;**60**:174-182. DOI: 10.1007/s00239-004-0046-3

[16] Bolotin A, Quinquis B, Sorokin A, Ehrlich SD. Clustered regularly interspaced short palindrome repeats (CRISPRs) have spacers of extrachromosomal origin. Microbiology. 2005;**151**:2551-2561. DOI: 10.1099/mic.0.28048-0

[17] Barrangou R, Fremaux C, Deveau H, Richards M, Boyaval P, Moineau S, et al. CRISPR provides acquired resistance against viruses in prokaryotes. Science. 2007;**315**:1709-1712. DOI: 10.1126/science.1138140

[18] Brouns SJ, Jore MM, Lundgren M, Westra ER, Slijkhuis RJ, Snijders AP, et al. Small CRISPR RNAs guide antiviral defense in prokaryotes. Science. 2008;**321**:960-964. DOI: 10.1126/science.1159689

[19] Westra ER, van Erp PB, Kunne T, Wong SP, Staals RH, Seegers CL, et al. CRISPR immunity relies on the consecutive binding and degradation of negatively supercoiled invader DNA by Cascade and Cas3. Molecular Cell. 2012;**46**:595-605. DOI: 10.1016/j.molcel.2012.03.018

[20] Cong L, Ran FA, Cox D, Lin S, Barretto R, Habib N, et al. Multiplex genome engineering using CRISPR/Cas systems. Science. 2013;**339**:819-823. DOI: 10.1126/science.1231143

[21] Mali P, Yang L, Esvelt KM, Aach J, Guell M, DiCarlo JE, et al. RNA-guided human genome engineering via Cas9. Science. 2013;**339**:823-826. DOI: 10.1126/science.1232033

[22] Karginov FV, Hannon GJ. The CRISPR system: Small RNA-guided defense in bacteria and archaea. Molecular Cell. 2010;**37**:7-19. DOI: 10.1016/j.molcel.2009.12.033

[23] Jore MM, Brouns SJ, van der Oost J. RNA in defense: CRISPRs protect prokaryotes against mobile genetic elements. Cold Spring Harbor Perspectives in Biology. 2012;**4**. DOI: 10.1101/cshperspect.a003657

[24] Louwen R, Staals RH, Endtz HP, van Baarlen P, van der Oost J. The role of CRISPR-Cas systems in virulence of pathogenic bacteria. Microbiology and Molecular Biology Reviews. 2014;**78**:74-88. DOI: 10.1128/MMBR.00039-13

[25] Hsu PD, Lander ES, Zhang F. Development and applications of CRISPR-Cas9 for genome engineering. Cell. 2014;**157**:1262-1278. DOI: 10.1016/j.cell.2014.05.010

[26] Ratner HK, Sampson TR, Weiss DS. Overview of CRISPR-Cas9 biology. Cold Spring Harbor Protocols. 2016;**2016**. DOI: 10.1101/pdb.top088849

[27] Adli M. The CRISPR tool kit for genome editing and beyond. Nature Communications. 2018;**9**:1911. DOI: 10.1038/s41467-018-04252-2

[28] Cheo DL, Titus SA, Byrd DR, Hartley JL, Temple GF, Brasch MA. Concerted assembly and cloning of multiple DNA segments using in vitro site-specific recombination: Functional analysis of multi-segment expression clones. Genome Research. 2004;**14**:2111-2120. DOI: 10.1101/gr.2512204

[29] Magnani E, Bartling L, Hake S. From Gateway to MultiSite Gateway in one recombination event. BMC Molecular Biology. 2006;**7**. DOI: 46. DOI: 10.1186/1471-2199-7-46

[30] Goodarzi AA, Jeggo PA. The repair and signaling responses to DNA double-strand breaks. Advances in Genetics. 2013;**82**:1-45. DOI: 10.1016/B978-0-12-407676-1.00001-9

[31] Beucher A, Birraux J, Tchouandong L, Barton O, Shibata A, Conrad S, et al. ATM and Artemis promote homologous recombination of radiation-induced DNA double-strand breaks in G2. The EMBO Journal. 2009;**28**:3413-3427. DOI: 10.1038/emboj.2009.276

[32] Rodgers K, McVey M. Error-prone repair of DNA double-strand breaks. Journal of Cellular Physiology. 2016;**231**:15-24. DOI: 10.1002/jcp.25053

[33] van Heemst D, Brugmans L, Verkaik NS, van Gent DC. End-joining of blunt DNA double-strand breaks in mammalian fibroblasts is precise and requires DNA-PK and XRCC4. DNA Repair. 2004;**3**:43-50

[34] Kuzminov A. Recombinational repair of DNA damage in *Escherichia coli* and bacteriophage lambda. Microbiology and Molecular Biology Reviews. 1999;**63**:751-813

[35] San Filippo J, Sung P, Klein H. Mechanism of eukaryotic homologous recombination. Annual Review of Biochemistry. 2008;**77**:229-257. DOI: 10.1146/annurev.biochem.77.061306.125255

[36] McVey M, Lee SE. MMEJ repair of double-strand breaks (director's cut): Deleted sequences and alternative endings. Trends in Genetics. 2008;**24**:529-538. DOI: 10.1016/j.tig.2008.08.007

[37] Sfeir A, Symington LS. Microhomology-mediated end joining: A back-up survival mechanism or dedicated pathway? Trends in Biochemical Sciences. 2015;**40**:701-714. DOI: 10.1016/j.tibs.2015.08.006

[38] Sinha S, Villarreal D, Shim EY, Lee SE. Risky business: Microhomology-mediated end joining. Mutation Research. 2016;**788**:17-24. DOI: 10.1016/j.mrfmmm.2015.12.005

[39] Seol JH, Shim EY, Lee SE. Microhomology-mediated end joining: Good, bad and ugly. Mutation Research. 2018;**809**:81-87. DOI: 10.1016/j.mrfmmm.2017.07.002

[40] Lander N, Chiurillo MA, Docampo R. Genome editing by CRISPR/Cas9: A game change in the genetic manipulation of protists. The Journal of Eukaryotic Microbiology. 2016;**63**:679-690. DOI: 10.1111/jeu.12338

[41] Vu GTH, Cao HX, Fauser F, Reiss B, Puchta H, Schubert I. Endogenous sequence patterns predispose the repair modes of CRISPR/Cas9-induced DNA double-stranded breaks in *Arabidopsis thaliana*. The Plant Journal. 2017;**92**:57-67. DOI: 10.1111/tpj.13634

[42] Nakade S, Tsubota T, Sakane Y, Kume S, Sakamoto N, Obara M, et al. Microhomology-mediated end-joining-dependent integration of donor DNA in cells and animals using TALENs and CRISPR/Cas9. Nature Communications. 2014;**5**:5560. DOI: 10.1038/ncomms6560

[43] Yao X, Wang X, Liu J, Hu X, Shi L, Shen X, et al. CRISPR/Cas9-mediated precise targeted integration *in vivo* using a double cut donor with short homology arms. eBioMedicine. 2017;**20**:19-26. DOI: 10.1016/j.ebiom.2017.05.015

[44] Sakuma T, Yamamoto T. Magic wands of CRISPR-lots of choices for gene knock-in. Cell Biology and Toxicology. 2017;**33**:501-505. DOI: 10.1016/j.ebiom.2017.05.015

[45] Dickinson DJ, Goldstein B. CRISPR-based methods for *Caenorhabditis elegans* genome engineering. Genetics. 2016;**202**:885-901. DOI: 10.1534/genetics.115.182162

[46] Paix A, Wang Y, Smith HE, Lee CY, Calidas D, Lu T, et al. Scalable and versatile genome editing using linear DNAs with microhomology to Cas9 Sites in *Caenorhabditis elegans*. Genetics. 2014;**198**:1347-1356. DOI: 10.1534/genetics.114.170423

[47] Sakuma T, Nakade S, Sakane Y, Suzuki KT, Yamamoto T. MMEJ-assisted gene knock-in using TALENs and CRISPR-Cas9 with the PITCh systems. Nature Protocols. 2016;**11**:118-133. DOI: 10.1038/nprot.2015.140

[48] Shy BR, MacDougall MS, Clarke R, Merrill BJ. Co-incident insertion enables high efficiency genome engineering in mouse embryonic stem cells. Nucleic Acids Research. 2016;**44**:7997-8010. DOI: 10.1093/nar/gkw685

[49] Dickinson DJ, Pani AM, Heppert JK, Higgins CD, Goldstein B. Streamlined genome engineering with a self-excising drug selection cassette. Genetics. 2015;**200**:1035-1049. DOI: 10.1534/genetics.115.178335

[50] Ruan J, Li H, Xu K, Wu T, Wei J, Zhou R, et al. Highly efficient CRISPR/Cas9-mediated transgene knockin at the H11 locus in pigs. Scientific Reports. 2015;**5**:14253. DOI: 10.1038/srep14253

[51] Zhang L, Jia R, Palange NJ, Satheka AC, Togo J, An Y, et al. Large genomic fragment deletions and insertions in mouse using CRISPR/Cas9. PLoS One. 2015;**10**:e0120396. DOI: 10.1371/journal.pone.0120396

[52] Yasuda T, Kagawa W, Ogi T, Kato TA, Suzuki T, Dohmae N, et al. Novel function of HATs and HDACs in homologous recombination through acetylation of human RAD52 at double-strand break sites. PLoS Genetics. 2018;**14**:e1007277. DOI: 10.1371/journal.pgen.1007277

[53] Yao X, Zhang M, Wang X, Ying W, Hu X, Dai P, et al. Tild-CRISPR allows for efficient and precise gene knockin in mouse and human cells. Developmental Cell. 2018;**45**:526, e525-536. DOI: 10.1016/j.devcel.2018.04.021

[54] Park J, Throop AL, LaBaer J. Site-specific recombinational cloning using gateway and in-fusion cloning schemes. Current Protocols in Molecular Biology. 2015;**110**(3):20 21-20 23. DOI: 10.1002/0471142727.mb0320s110

[55] Kime C, Mandegar MA, Srivastava D, Yamanaka S, Conklin BR, Rand TA. Efficient CRISPR/Cas9-based genome engineering in human pluripotent stem cells. Current Protocols in Human Genetics. 2016;**88**(21):24. DOI: 10.1002/0471142905.hg2104s88

[56] Hartley JL, Temple GF, Brasch MA. DNA cloning using *in vitro* site-specific recombination. Genome Research. 2000;**10**:1788-1795

[57] Landy A. Dynamic, structural, and regulatory aspects of lambda site-specific recombination. Annual Review of Biochemistry. 1989;**58**:913-949. DOI: 10.1146/annurev.bi.58.070189.004405

[58] Ogura T, Hiraga S. Mini-F plasmid genes that couple host cell division to plasmid proliferation. Proceedings of the National Academy of Sciences of the United States of America. 1983;**80**:4784-4788

[59] Bernard P, Couturier M. Cell killing by the F plasmid CcdB protein involves poisoning of DNA-topoisomerase II complexes. Journal of Molecular Biology. 1992;**226**:735-745

[60] Bernard P, Kezdy KE, Van Melderen L, Steyaert J, Wyns L, Pato ML, et al. The F plasmid CcdB protein induces efficient ATP-dependent DNA cleavage by gyrase. Journal of Molecular Biology. 1993;**234**:534-541. DOI: 10.1006/jmbi.1993.1609

[61] Bahassi EM, O'Dea MH, Allali N, Messens J, Gellert M, Couturier M. Interactions of CcdB with DNA gyrase. Inactivation of Gyra, poisoning of the gyrase-DNA complex, and the antidote action of CcdA. The Journal of Biological Chemistry. 1999;**274**:10936-10944

[62] Petersen LK, Stowers RS. A Gateway MultiSite recombination cloning toolkit. PLoS One. 2011;**6**:e24531. DOI: 10.1371/journal.pone.0024531

[63] Sasaki Y, Sone T, Yoshida S, Yahata K, Hotta J, Chesnut JD, et al. Evidence for high specificity and efficiency of multiple recombination signals in mixed DNA cloning by the Multisite Gateway system. Journal of Bacteriology. 2004;**107**:233-243

[64] Stark JM, Pierce AJ, Oh J, Pastink A, Jasin M. Genetic steps of mammalian homologous repair with distinct mutagenic consequences. Molecular and Cellular Biology. 2004;**24**:9305-9316. DOI: 10.1128/MCB.24.21.9305-9316.2004

[65] Maruyama T, Dougan SK, Truttmann MC, Bilate AM, Ingram JR, Ploegh HL. Increasing the efficiency of precise genome editing with CRISPR-Cas9 by inhibition of nonhomologous end joining. Nature Biotechnology. 2015;**33**:538-542. DOI: 10.1038/nbt.3190

[66] Chu VT, Weber T, Wefers B, Wurst W, Sander S, Rajewsky K, et al. Increasing the efficiency of homology-directed repair for CRISPR-Cas9-induced precise gene editing in mammalian cells. Nature Biotechnology. 2015;**33**:543-548. DOI: 10.1038/nbt.3198

[67] Vartak SV, Raghavan SC. Inhibition of nonhomologous end joining to increase the specificity of CRISPR/Cas9 genome editing. The FEBS Journal. 2015;**282**:4289-4294. DOI: 10.1111/febs.13416

[68] Li G, Zhang X, Zhong C, Mo J, Quan R, Yang J, et al. Small molecules enhance CRISPR/Cas9-mediated homology-directed genome editing in primary cells. Scientific Reports. 2017;**7**:8943. DOI: 10.1038/s41598-017-09306-x

[69] Srivastava M, Nambiar M, Sharma S, Karki SS, Goldsmith G, Hegde M, et al. An inhibitor of nonhomologous end-joining abrogates double-strand break repair and impedes cancer progression. Cell. 2012;**151**:1474-1487. DOI: 10.1016/j.cell.2012.11.054

[70] Yu C, Liu Y, Ma T, Liu K, Xu S, Zhang Y, et al. Small molecules enhance CRISPR genome editing in pluripotent stem cells. Cell Stem Cell. 2015;**16**:142-147. DOI: 10.1016/j.stem.2015.01.003

Chapter 7

Machine Learning and Rule Mining Techniques in the Study of Gene Inactivation and RNA Interference

Saurav Mallik, Ujjwal Maulik, Namrata Tomar,
Tapas Bhadra, Anirban Mukhopadhyay and
Ayan Mukherji

Additional information is available at the end of the chapter

http://dx.doi.org/10.5772/intechopen.83470

Abstract

RNA interference (RNAi) and gene inactivation are extensively used biological terms in biomedical research. Two categories of small ribonucleic acid (RNA) molecules, *viz.*, microRNA (miRNA) and small interfering RNA (siRNA) are central to the RNAi. There are various kinds of algorithms developed related to RNAi and gene silencing. In this book chapter, we provided a comprehensive review of various machine learning and association rule mining algorithms developed to handle different biological problems such as detection of gene signature, biomarker, gene module, potentially disordered protein, differentially methylated region and many more. We also provided a comparative study of different well-known classifiers along with other used methods. In addition, we demonstrated the brief biological information regarding the immense biological challenges for gene activation as well as their advantages, disadvantages and possible therapeutic strategies. Finally, our study helps the bioinformaticians to understand the overall immense idea in different research dimensions including several learning algorithms for the benevolent of the disease discovery.

Keywords: machine learning, association rule mining, RNAi, gene silencing, multi-omics data

1. Introduction

RNAi [1] is an innate biological process in which RNA molecules inhibit gene expression or translation [2] by suppressing targeted mRNA molecules. Since the discovery of RNAi by

Andrew Fire and Craig Mello, it has become evident that RNAi has immense potential in suppression of desired genes [3]. The first evidence that double-stranded RNA (dsRNA) could achieve efficient gene silencing through RNAi came from studies on the nematode *Caenorhabditis elegans* [4] and *Drosophila melanogaster* [5], which lead toward understanding the biochemical nature of the RNAi pathway. Two types of small ribonucleic acid (RNA) molecules—microRNA (miRNA) and small interfering RNA (siRNA)—are central to RNAi [6]. To compare two types of elicit RNAi, the siRNA must be fully complementary to its target mRNA, whereas, miRNA only needs to be partially complementary to its target mRNA. In organisms like *C. elegans* and *D. melanogaster*, RNAi can be induced by introducing long dsRNA complementary to the target mRNA to be degraded, however, in mammalian cells and organisms, introducing dsRNA longer than 30 bp activates a potent antiviral response. To solve this limitation, siRNAs are used to induce RNAi in mammalian cells and organisms [7–9].

The discovery of both siRNA and miRNA provides a new therapeutic approach [10, 11] for the treatment of diseases by targeting genes that have undesired mutated or overexpression of normal genes. The RNAi Process is as following. SiRNAs that induce the degradation of specific endogenous is very common phenomenon in eukaryotic cells to inhibit protein production at post transcriptional level [12]. The RNAi process is initiated by short dsRNAs, 21–25 nucleotides that lead to the sequence specific inhibition of their homologous mRNAs. These siRNAs are normally produced in cells from cleavage of longer dsRNA precursors by Dicer that is a ribonuclease III family member. The cleaved parts are incorporated into a multicomponent nuclease complex known as the RNA-induced silencing complexes (RISC), which contain the splicing protein Argonaute-2 (Ago-2) [13]. The ssRNA derived from the short dsRNA acts as a antisense strand directing the complex to the specific target mRNA; in where a RISC-associated endoribonuclease cleavages the target mRNA [14]. Therapeutic approaches based on siRNA involve the introduction of a synthetic siRNA into the target cells to elicit RNAi, thereby inhibiting the expression of a specific messenger RNA (mRNA) to produce a gene silencing effect [15]. RNAi is beneficial in accelerating cures in medicine, especially when a disease is thought to due to a defective gene [16]. For historical perspective, the first application of RNAi therapy was in age-related macular degeneration (AMD) by using siRNAs to suppress the vascular endothelial growth factor (VEGF) pathway that causes abnormal growth of blood vessels behind the retina, carried out directly to the patient's eye [17]. RNAi techniques have been used against the spread of tumor growth and increasing its sensitization toward drug treatment, RNAi technology will be beneficial to selectively affect cancer cells without damaging normal cells as the RNAi therapy against cancer cells is used for directly targeting the oncogenes; and therefore, found to stop progression and invasion of the tumor cells [18, 19] and also increase the sensitization of tumor against drug, as mentioned earlier [20]. As RNAi can silence disease-associated genes in tissue culture and animal models, the development of RNAi-based reagents for therapeutic applications involves technological enhancements that improve siRNA stability and delivery *in vivo* [21], while minimizing off-target and nonspecific effects.

A number of different approaches have been developed for the *in vivo* delivery of siRNA, among which, rapid infusion by hydrodynamic injection of siRNA achieves the best delivery in rodents [22]. However, this way, the delivery is restricted to highly vascularized tissues, such as the liver [23] and also, it is currently not a viable method for delivery in human clinical studies. Lipid-based *in vivo* applications have been devised [24], which have been used extensively for cell culture experiments, with some issues, like the cationic nature of the lipids used in cell culture leads to aggregation when used in animals and results in rapid serum clearance and lung accumulation. Even then, there are an increasing number of reports citing success with lipid-mediated delivery of siRNAs *in vivo*. To improve the delivery of siRNA into human liver cells [25] without transfection agents, lipophilic siRNAs were conjugated with derivatives of cholesterol, lithocholic acid, or lauric acid, where the lipid moieties were covalently linked to the 5′-ends of the RNAs using phosphoramidite chemistry [26]. These could down-regulate the expression of a LacZ expression construct. By conjugating cholesterol to the 3′-end of the sense strand of siRNA by means of a pyrrolidine linker, the pharmacological properties of siRNA molecules was improved by Soutschek et al. [27]. Advantages of cholesterol attachments are evident as being more resistant to nuclease degradation, more stable in the blood by increasing binding to human serum albumin and increased uptake of siRNA molecules by the liver. Intravascular delivery of siRNA molecules is a very simple technique, which was used to protect mice from fulminant hepatitis using siRNAs against Fas receptors by Song et al. [28], who administer Fas siRNA by intravenous injection into mice over a 24-hour period. The authors could show the persist effects for 10 days and protected mice against experimentally induced liver fibrosis. Local delivery of siRNAs have also been tried into the eye to target the VEGF pathway and shown that it could be therapeutically beneficial in neovascularization-related eye diseases. SiRNA topical gels have also been used to deliver them to cells in dermatological applications and cervical cancer treatment [29]. Gene gun method was used for an intradermal administration of nucleic acids to enhance cancer vaccine potency [30]. The other technique is an electroporation, which has been used to deliver siRNAs into the brain [31] and muscles of rodents. Injecting viral vectors for the *in vivo* delivery of siRNA directly have been tried, where an adeno-associated virus (AAV) associated shRNA vector injected directly into the midbrain neurons of adult mice to silence of the tyrosine hydroxylase gene near the site of injection for several weeks. However, there exist an alternative to injection, called as an *ex vivo* approach to generate human immunodeficiency virus (HIV)-1-resistant lymphocytes and macrophages [32]. It was accomplished through using a lentiviral vector, an anti-rev siRNA construct into CD34(+) hematopoietic progenitor cells. The siRNA-transduced progenitor cells were allowed to mature into macrophages *in vitro* and T-cells *in vivo*, [33].

Many machine learning, bio-statistical [34] and association rule mining methods [35] are available that have been developed to solve different problems related to gene silencing and disease discovery. In this book chapter, we provided a comprehensive survey of different machine learning and association rule mining algorithms developed for tackling various biological challenges such as detection of gene signature, biomarker, gene module, potentially disordered protein detection, differentially methylated region, multi-omics data integration, etc. We also described a comparative study of different well-known classifiers along with other used methods for the study. Meanwhile, many gene module discovery based approaches are also developed that employs several machine learning, deep learning and soft computing approaches. In addition, many multi-objective algorithms are also developed to find optimal multi-omics genetic signatures for the respective disease. Furthermore, we demonstrated the

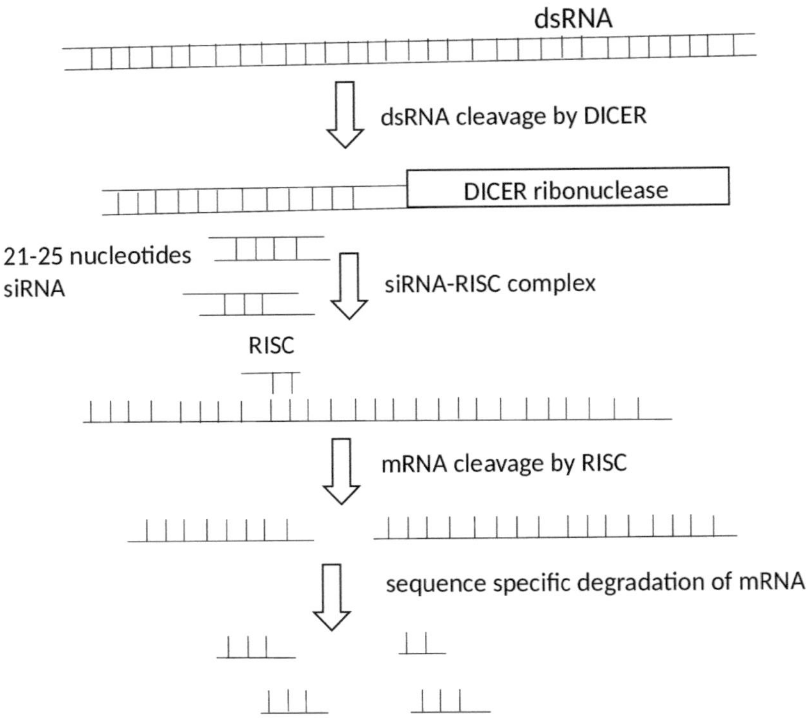

Figure 1. Flowchart of the RNAi mechanism [37, 38].

brief biological information regarding the immense biological challenges for gene activation and their advantages, disadvantages and possible therapeutic strategies. There are certain challenges exist, such as off-target effects, cytotoxicity, need for efficient delivery methods, their clinical implementation need efficient delivery vehicles and siRNA activity, itself, non-specific gene silencing, activation of innate immune system, the lack of efficient in vivo delivery systems still remain to be handled. Apart from these challenges, the development of efficient tissue-specific and differentiation dependent expression of siRNA is essential for transgenic and therapeutic approaches. However, there are successful *in vitro* and *in vivo* experiments for raising hopes in treating human diseases with RNAi [36]. Moreover, our study is useful for the researchers to understand the central idea about RNAi and gene silencing, along with the current machine/deep learning and association rule mining algorithms related to these (**Figure 1**).

2. Fundamental concepts

In this section, some basic symbols of the graph mining, pattern recognition, [39] and information theory are described. A graph is an ordered pair G = (V, E) comprising of a set of vertices denoted as V and a set of edges denoted as E. To avoid ambiguity, the graph is described here precisely as undirected and simple. Let, $Q = (N, E)$ be an unweighted as well as undirected

http://dx.doi.org/10.5772/intechopen.83470

graph, and H be a (hypograph) of it, ($H \subseteq N$). Further, suppose, the density of H, denoted by $Ds(H)$, be defined as $Ds(H) = \frac{|IE(H)|}{|H|}$, where $IE(H)$ depicts the induced edge-set of H, and $|H|$ refers to the cardinality of H. Suppose, the highest density of the graph H, referred to as $Ds^*(H)$, is illustrated as follows: $Ds^*(H) = \max_{H \subseteq V}\{DS(H)\}$. Now, if $Q = (N, E)$ is a weighted graph, $Ds(H)$ will be $\frac{\sum_{e \in IE(H)} wt_e}{|H|}$, where $IE(H)$ symbolizes the induced edge-set of H, and wt_e denotes the weight of the edge $e \in IE(H)$. Entropy of a random variable evaluates the amount of uncertainty corresponding to the variable [40]. The entropy of a discrete variable A, referred to as $EP(A)$, is defined in the following: $EP(A) = -\sum_{a \in A} p(a) \log_b p(a)$, where $p(a)$ refers to the probability mass function of A, and the value of b, in general, is considered as 2. Mutual information [41] between two random variables estimates the quantity of information that they combinedly share, i.e., the mutual dependency between them. When mutual information is zero, this signifies that these two variables are entirely independent to each other; whereas when mutual information is higher, it signifies that these two variables are extremely dependent on each other.

Topological Overlap Measure (TOM) and other related measures: Ravasz et al. [42] proposed a new measure Topological Overlap Measure (TOM) that provided the similarity between two nodes belonging to a network depending upon nearest neighbor concept. Furthermore, various modified versions of TOM such as weighted TOM (wTOM) [43], generalized TOM (GTOM) [44] are present in the literature. In the course of computing the wTOM, Pearson correlation coefficient scores are first evaluated for all pairs of vertices, and then a soft thresholding power (say, $\beta >= 1$) is utilized from the correlation coefficient matrix through scale free topology. After that, weighted adjacency matrix is calculated using the coefficient matrix using the calculated power β. Then wTOM is computed from the weighted adjacency matrix. In the same way, the GTOM can also be defined just like TOM except it counts the number of m-step neighbors while calculating TOM measure between two vertices. Now, for calculating GTOM of order 0 (i.e., GTOM0), the adjacency score becomes the score of GTOM0. But, for determining the GTOM with higher order than zero (i.e., GTOM1, GTOM2, GTOM3,...), it follows the same procedure of TOM calculation, but counts up to $\ddot{d}$-th neighbors for each vertex ($\ddot{d} = 1, 2, 3, \ldots$). Notably, GTOM1, GTOM2 and other higher order GTOM work only on binary matrix. So, before using those measures, the weighted adjacency matrix is translated into binary matrix in which the greater adjacency value than a specified cutoff (e.g., 70% score of the distance between the minimum and maximum adjacency values is converted into 1, and the lower value than the cutoff is transferred into 0.

In data mining, hierarchical clustering is one of the most popular cluster analyses in forming a hierarchy of clusters. There exist two types of strategies: agglomerative and divisive [45]. As is already known, agglomerative hierarchical clustering does not need any input parameters except the similarity matrix. Thus, there is no extra burden of utilizing cluster initialization as it simply merges two closest clusters at each iteration and continues till a singleton cluster is found. Divisive hierarchical clustering also follows the same style but in a reverse order. This is the major benefit of performing hierarchical clustering over the traditional K-means clustering algorithm, which is sensitive to initialization.

Association rule mining (ARM) [46] is a popular method for generating interesting relationships among different items (*viz.*, genes). Suppose, $GST = \{g_1, g_2, \ldots, g_n\}$ be a item set (gene set) and $SST = \{s_1, s_2, \ldots, s_m\}$ be sample set (*viz.*, transaction set). Therefore, an association rule can be stated as $A \Rightarrow C$, where $A, C \subseteq GST$ and $A \cap C = \phi$. Notably, A and C symbolize as antecedent and consequent, respectively. An association rule can be described as the cause-effect relationships of the corresponding item sets in the transactions of a transactional data-profile in a big shopping market. A set of bought items may fall into a transaction. In a similar fashion, many genes may occur together in a sample (transaction) of a gene expression profile or similar profile. Many of these genes may be up-regulated or down-regulated, whereas the remaining genes will be non-differentially expressed.

3. Machine learning and rule mining approaches for gene inactivation

Currently, omics data analysis is one of the widely popular research domains. It can be categorized into two major types, single-omics data analysis, and multi-omics data analysis. In earlier, single-omics data processing such as gene expression data processing was highly popular. In those days, basically microarray gene expression data was popular. Now, the microarray data becomes obsolete while RNAseq, next-generation sequencing (NGS) and whole exome sequencing (WES) data become popular. However, the major aim of the single omics data analysis was to identify genetic marker as well as gene module identification. In current era, multi-omics data integration is now a big challenge to any researcher since it consists of various kind of profiles that are either proportional or inversely proportional to each other. Different kinds of regression analysis (logistic regression, sglasso [47, 48], flasso [47], etc.) are popular to integrate the multi-omics data. In case of the multi-omics data, the aim is to determine either single (or, combinatorial) gene marker, or gene signature, or multi-biomolecular closed bio-circuit. There are many machine learning and association rule mining methods available that have been developed to solve different problems related to gene silencing and disease discovery (**Table 1** for tools and **Table 2** for their application). For this regard, Bandyopadhyay et al. provided a comprehensive survey of various statistical tests for determining differentially expressed transcripts from microarray or other related datasets [69]. Then a rank based weighted association rule mining, RANWAR is developed to identify weighted interesting genomic rules applicable to any kind of genomic or epigenomic data [9]. A new technique of gene-based association rule mining approach was developed in [62]. Next, another statistics-based association rule mining technique "StatBicRM" had been proposed that utilized statistical test and Binary Inclusion maximal algorithm (BiMax) to find classification-based genetic rules [46]. Reverently, further enhancement of "StatBicRM" algorithm was performed and a new method of combinatorial marker discovery had been developed whose central concept was based upon the inverse relationship between the gene expression and methylation pattern [50]. In addition, mutual information based feature selection strategy had been incorporated into the statistical methodology, and a new method of identifying epigenetic biomarkers through maximal relevance and minimal redundancy based feature (gene) selection method from bi-omics dataset was proposed [63]. A new method of

Method name	Reference	Type	Brief description
Multi-view gene modules using hypograph mining	Bhadra et al. [49]	Gene-module detection	Module detection from multi-view data using the statistical test and mutual information based dense subgraph.
RANWAR	Mallik et al. [9]	Rank based genomic rule mining	Rank based weighted association rule mining to identify interesting genomic rules applicable to any genomic/epigenomic data.
Combinatorial marker discovery by integrating multiple profiles	Bandyopadhyay et al. [50]	Combinatorial marker discovery	Integrating gene expression and methylation profiles, and identifying combinatorial gene markers.
DTFP-growth	Mallik et al. [51]	Gene based ARM	Multiple-threshold based ARM integrating gene expression, methylation and protein-protein interaction profiles.
StatBicRM	Maulik et al. [46]	Statistical biclustering-based rule mining	Statistical biclustering-based rule mining and analyzing the gene expression and methylation data profiles using it.
sglasso	Augugliaro [47, 48]	Regression method	Sglasso tool develops the structured graphical lasso estimator for the weighted l1-penalized RCON(V, E) model.
flasso	Augugliaro [47, 52]	Regression method	Implements the weight l1-penlized factorial dynamic Gaussian graphical model.
MVDA	Serra et al. [53]	Multi-view genomic profile integration	Works to conjoin the those kinds of data at the levels of the outcomes of every single view clustering iteration.
Machine learning for epigenetics and future medical applications	Holder et al. [54]	Machine learning and deep learning approaches	Active learning and imbalanced class learning are utilized to solve the shortcoming with machine learning for building better feature selection and solving the imbalance data problem.
A machine learning approach to integrate big data for precision medicine	Lee et al. [55]	Molecular marker discovery	The robust molecular markers that might be useful for targeted treatment of the acute myeloid leukemia are identified.
Deep learning based multi-omics integration robustly predicts survival	Chaudhary et al. [56]	Deep learning based multi-omics integration method	A deep learning method is used to integrate multi-omics data and to perform survival study on hepatocellular carcinoma.
Deep learning for genomics: a concise overview	Yue et al. [57]	Deep learning applications on genomic data	The strengths of various deep learning methodologies are demonstrated that are applicable on any kind of genomic profile.
intNMF	Chalise and Fridley [58]	Integrative clustering method	Integrative clustering of several high dimensional profiles and subtype classification by non-negative matrix factorization (NMF).
Multi-modal data analysis for heterogeneous data	Yang and Michailidis [59]	Module detection for heterogeneous data	The multi-modal profile analysis is conducted for heterogeneous data depending upon NMF.
Comparative study and evaluation of the integrative techniques for the multilevel omics data	Pucher et al. [60]	Integrative method for multilevel omics profiles	The comparative study of three integrative methods (*viz.*, NMF, sparse canonical correlation analysis (sCCA) and logic data mining MicroArray Logic Analyzer

Method name	Reference	Type	Brief description
			(MALA)) is conducted on simulated data and real omics profile.
WeCoMXP	Mallik and Bandyopadhyay [61]	Weighted connectivity (similarity) measure	*WeCoMXP* is developed integrating co-expression, co-methylation and protein-protein interactions, and useful for determining the similarity between any two molecules.
Tumor prediction using integrated analysis of expression and methylation	Mallik et al. [62]	Rule-based classifier	Integrated analysis of gene expression and DNA methylation and classification rule mining for tumor/cancer prediction.
Epigenetic gene marker discovery through feature selection	Mallik et al. [63]	Gene based ARM	Epigenetic gene marker discovery using maximal relevance and minimal redundancy based feature selection.

Table 1. The machine learning and rule mining methods related to gene inactivation and RNAi.

Method name	Reference	Type	Brief description
TF-MiRNA-gene network based modules for cytosine variants	Sen et al. [64]	Module detection	TF-MiRNA-gene network based module detection for 5hmC and 5mC brain samples between human and rhesus.
IDPT	Mallik et al. [65]	Intrinsically disordered protein finding	Potential intrinsically disordered protein identification through transcriptomic analysis of genes for epigenetic data.
Integration of DNA methylation data and gene expression data	Singh et al. [66]	Finding differentially methylated regions	Differentially methylated regions are determined and further statistical analysis is performed.
Application of machine-learning algorithms for gene expression regulation	Cheng and Worzel [67]	Applications of machine learning methods on gene regulation	The machine learning strategies on gene regulation are reviewed, and their functional links mediated by histone modifications and transcription factors are demonstrated.
Application of machine-learning techniques on histone methylation	Xu et al. [68]	Predictive model of gene expression by epigenetic factors by regression	A new model is developed to predict the gene expression using the function of histone modification levels through multi-linear regression multivariate adaptive regression splines.

Table 2. Applications of machine learning and rule mining methods related to gene inactivation.

identifying multi-view gene-module identification was also proposed that applied the integrated methodology of statistical method and dense subgraph mining [49]. Detection of strongly connected genetic modules in multi-omics regulatory networks is an important study for the integrated study analysis of the network-based architecture. Many profiles belonging to the multi-omics datasets basically consist of a massive amount of genes, many of them are noisy and redundant. Such kind of noisy and redundant genes (or, features) are irrelevant while obtaining knowledge from the data. Furthermore, it is computationally absurd to utilize any clustering technique on such type of huge sized data profiles to get the dense genetic clusters. In many times, researchers face problems while calculating and subsequently accumulating the similarity matrix of such massive dimensions consisting of all the mutual dependency information between all the possible gene-pairs equivalent to every such profile. So, managing the high dimensionality of the underlying profile is a critical challenge to the researchers. To overcome the "curse of dimensionality" problem, the job of feature selection is basically treated as one of the most important preprocessing works to remove such noisy and redundant genes, which in turn decreases the total elapsed time. The main purpose of the feature selection is to find an optimal subset of features depending on some optimization conditions by which efficient knowledge discovery can be performed [70]. Depending on the availability of the class labels, the feature selection process can be organized into two types: supervised and unsupervised [71]. Unsupervised feature selection does not need the class label information while choosing the minimized feature subset [72], whereas supervised feature selection selects a subset of favorable features by utilizing the knowledge of class labels into the feature selection procedure. In the case of supervised feature selection, significant test [73], mutual information [74], are some broadly used measures to evaluate the excellence of the candidate features. In the territory of biological rematches, a statistical test is generally treated as one of the important tools for obtaining the significant genes for the big sized datasets, and therefore aids in decreasing the size of the dataset. There are different types of statistical tests such as t-test, significant analysis of microarrays, empirical Bayes test, etc. in the literature.

The significant genes therefore provide a weighted graph in which the nodes refer to the significant genes and the weighted edges signify the association between the related two nodes. Recently, graph data can be obtained in different rising fields of studies for forming the complicated structures *viz.*, biological networks, chemical compounds, social networks, protein structures, etc. With the increasing stipulate on the analysis of large sized structured data, graph mining has become one of the most demanding topics of research for identifying the critical relationships among various entities included in the large graphs [75]. In the recent era, analyzing multi-omics dataset is one of the emerging topics of research where different profiles denoting several directions are applied to carry out different important tasks *viz.*, marker determination, classification, and clustering. For this regard, many research works have been performed in the following directions *viz.*, marker identification [76], classification [77], clustering [78], etc. Recently, Bhadra et al. [49] have developed a new algorithm handling an integrated study comprising of statistical method and normalized mutual information oriented hypo-graph mining to find the multi-omics co-similar genetic modules present in multi-omics datasets. Formerly, various statistical (*viz.*, correlation, regression oriented) and/or weight-based techniques (*viz.*, [79]) are matured for multi-omics data integration, but not for multi-omics genetic-module detecting. Furthermore, some multi-view data integration mechanism employs various soft-computing methods such as clustering, non-matrix factorization, etc. Recently, Serra et al. [53] proposed a framework for combining different data profiles of multi-view datasets by integrating several clustering results done on each profile through non-matrix factorization. Pucher et al. [60] provided a comprehensive review and comparative study of the three integrative methods (*viz.*, non-negative matrix factorization (NMF), sparse canonical correlation analysis (sCCA) and logic data mining MicroArray Logic Analyzer (MALA)) on simulated data as well as real omics profile. In addition, there are many deep

C4.5 classifier	K-nearest neighbors (KNN) classifier	Naive Bayes classifier	Support vector machines (SVM) classifier	Artificial neural networks (ANN) classifier
• Can use both discrete and continuous values.	• Can use only continuous values.	• Can use both discrete and continuous values.	• Can use only continuous values.	• Can use both discrete and continuous values.
• Handles noise.	• Sensitive to noisy features.	• Sensitive to noisy features.	• Is less effective when data contains noisy features.	• Handles noisy features.
• Classes need not be linearly separable.	• Classes need not be linearly separable.	• Classes need not be linearly separable.	• Works well even if data is not linearly separable in the input feature space.	• Works fine even if data is not linearly separable in the input feature space.
• Faces the problem of overfitting.	• Overcomes the problem of overfitting.	• Faces the problem of overfitting.	• Overcomes the problem of overfitting.	• Overcomes the problem of overfitting.
• Needs large searching time.	• Requires higher searching time for a larger data.	• Enormous Computational efficiency.	• Needs higher searching time for a larger data.	• Needs high processing time if neural network is huge.

Table 3. Comparison of different classifiers.

learning techniques that were also developed to handle biological data. Chaudhary et al. [56] proposed a deep learning based methodology to integrate multi-omics data and robustly perform survival study on hepatocellular carcinoma. Furthermore, there are many interesting applications of the above machine learning and deep learning techniques. For example, Xu et al. [68] developed a new model using the regression to predict the gene expression using the function of histone modifications/variants levels through the consecutive regression methods (*viz.*, multi-linear regression as well as multivariate adaptive regression splines). Mallik et al. [65] performed a comprehensive analysis to identify potential intrinsically disordered proteins through the transcriptomic analysis of genes for the expression and methylation data. To find differentially methylated regions is also an area of interest. Comparison of different classifiers used in many tools related to RNAi and gene inactivation is described in **Table 3**.

4. Biological challenges for gene inactivation

There are certain challenges exist, such as off-target effects, cytotoxicity, need for efficient delivery methods, their clinical implementation need efficient delivery vehicles and siRNA activity, itself, non-specific gene silencing, activation of innate immune system, the lack of efficient *in vivo* delivery systems still remain to be handled [80]. The effective delivery of RNAi therapeutics *in vivo* is one of the important challenge and have to consider several parameters for an efficient silencing, particle sizing, duration of the RNAi effect, its stability and modification, the delivery system and clearing off-target effects [81]. Apart from these challenges, the development of efficient tissue-specific and differentiation dependent expression of siRNA is essential for transgenic and therapeutic approaches. Bioactive drugs have been shown to perturb the naturally running system as these can clog/saturate the biochemical pathways. Since siRNA/shRNA relies on the endogenous microRNA machinery, thereby high doses of ectopic RNA have the risk of saturating all component of the miRNA pathway components. This was observed in the work by Grimm et al. [82] observed fatality association with high doses of liver-directed AAV-encoded shRNAs in mice, where high doses killed the recipient mice within 2 months. The length threshold of siRNAs seems to vary among cell types and it is an important consideration as dsRNA would induce innate immune responses that would eventually lead to cell death in mammalian. However, dsRNA less than 30 nucleotides have been shown good enough for no induction of cellular toxicity in mammalian and longer dsRNA is known to rapidly induce interferon responses. This suggests the careful risk assessment strategies when using longer and more potent Dicer substrates siRNAs. Moreover, correct RNAi targets are must, though ideal specificity of RNAi targets has not been shown. However if RNAi is going to silence off-targets, it can alter the gene function, which is clearly undesirable, therefore, care should be taken before-hand not to suppress the off-targets. If one third of siRNA are chosen randomly that it results in a toxic phenotype [83]. Comparison of siRNA and miRNA is described **Table 4**. However, there are successful *in vitro* and *in vivo* experiments for raising hopes in treating human disease with RNAi. The epigenetic network is one of the complex regulatory networks where epigenetic mechanisms such as DNA

siRNA	miRNA
• Must be fully complementary to its target mRNA.	• Can be partially complementary to its target mRNA.
• 21–23 nucleotide RNA duplex, notably endogenous siRNAs' origin is more polemic.	• 19–25 nucleotide RNA duplex, derived from gene units.
• dsRNA (30–100 nucleotides), before Dicer processing.	• Precursor miRNA (70–100 nucleotides) with interspersed mismatches and hairpin structure, prior to Dicer processing.
• One mRNA target.	• Can have multiple targets (>100 at the same time).
• For gene regulation, endonucleolytic cleavage of mRNA occurs.	• For gene regulation, translational repression degradation of mRNA occurs.
• Used as a therapeutic agent.	• Utility as a drug target therapeutic agent Diagnostic and biomarker tool.
• siRNAs shut down gene expression at a post-transcriptional level through mRNA degradation.	• MiRNAs silence their target genes mainly and most of the times through translational repression.
• Occurs in plants and lower animals, occurrence in mammals is questionable.	• Occurrence in plants and animals.
• Rarely found as an evolutionary conserved.	• Evolutionary conserved most of the time in the related organism.

Table 4. Comparison of siRNA and miRNA.

Disadvantages	Advantages and possible therapeutic strategies
• RNAi-based therapeutics has led to trigger several off-target (unintended) effects and hence shown host innate immune responses.	• Strategies for selective internalization and with endogenous mechanism without disrupting the natural pathway should be used to achieve maximal benefit from RNAi-based therapeutics.
• Pol III expressed shRNAs delivered in an AAV delivered in mice tail vein through injection was lethal due to acute liver failure.	• Levels of ectopic expression of therapeutic shRNAs should be carefully controlled (low yet effective) to avoid off target effects.
• Using naked siRNA has poor cellular uptake, it activates toll-like receptors and does not target to specific cell types.	• Naked siRNA are comparatively stable and non-immunogenic.
• Viral vectors for shRNA, expensive to create and cause immune reactions.	• High affinity toward infecting target cells, expression can long last.
• Lack of efficient delivery systems is the most critical challenge for the therapeutic applications of small RNAs.	• Identify the critical problem from the literature and allow researchers to publish failed ideas.

Table 5. Disadvantages, advantages of RNAi and possible therapeutic strategies.

methylation and modifications to histone proteins regulate gene expression and high-order DNA structure [84]. Epigenetics is basically a study of heritable changes in phenotypes where the DNA sequences are not changed anymore. DNA methylation [85] is an epigenetic factor that represents the inclusion of a methyl group (–CH3) to the fifth position of a cytosine pyrimidine ring or to the sixth nitrogen position of an adenine purine ring in genomic DNA. DNA methylation generally decreases belong to the gene expression level. In this connection, copy number variation (*CNV*) [86] is another latest domain of research in genomics. It is basically an event where the repetition of different portions of the genome continuously happens, and an alteration on the number of repeats in the genome is recognized between individual to individual in the human population. Copy number variation is a category of structural changes, especially, it is a type of either duplication or deletion event which generally influences a reasonable number of base pairs. It has been realized from recent researches that around two-thirds of the total human genome is made up of repeats. In the case of mammals, copy number alteration provides a significant contribution on producing the necessary deviation in both the population and disease phenotype. Cancer forms by various types of somatic genetic changes including copy-number alternations which affect the activity of the critical genes regulating the growth of the cell. Disadvantages and advantages of RNAi, and possible overcome strategies are demonstrated briefly in **Table 5**.

5. Conclusion

RNAi and gene inactivation are well-known research topics in the research of biomedical field. MiRNA and siRNA are closely associated with RNAi. Various categories of algorithms associated with RNAi and gene silencing have been developed in last 2 decades. In this book chapter, we provided a comprehensive review of various machine/deep learning as well as association rule mining algorithms that have been developed for handling different biological problems such as gene signature detection, multi-omics data integration, single/combinatorial biomarker identification, gene module detection, potentially disordered protein detection, differentially methylated region finding, and many more. Thereafter, a comparative study of several well-known classifiers along with other used approaches for the study has been included. In addition, we provided a brief biological description of the immense biological challenges for the gene activation along with their advantages, disadvantages and possible therapeutic strategies. Finally, this chapter helps the bioinformaticians to understand the central idea of RNAi and gene silencing along with their peripheral machine/deep learning and association rule mining algorithms for the benevolent of the disease discovery as well as possible therapeutic values.

Author details

Saurav Mallik[1,2]*, Ujjwal Maulik[3], Namrata Tomar[4], Tapas Bhadra[5], Anirban Mukhopadhyay[6] and Ayan Mukherji[7]

*Address all correspondence to: sauravmtech2@gmail.com

1 Machine Intelligence Unit, Indian Statistical Institute, Kolkata, India

2 Department of BioStatistics, University of Miami, Miami, Florida, USA

3 Department of Computer Science and Engineering, Jadavpur University, Kolkata, India

4 Department of Bio Medical Engineering, Medical College of Wisconsin, Milwaukee, WI, USA

5 Department of Computer Science and Engineering, Aliah University, Kolkata, India

6 Department of Computer Science and Engineering, University of Kalyani, Kalyani, West Bengal, India

7 Department of Computer Science and Engineering, Mallabhum Institute of Technology, Bishnupur, West Bengal, India

References

[1] Schwarz DS, Hutvagner G, Du T, Xu Z, Aronin N, et al. Asymmetry in the assembly of the RNAi enzyme complex. Cell. 2003;**115**(2):199-208

[2] van Dam S, Vosa U, van der Graaf A, Franke L, de Magalhes JP. Gene co-expression analysis for functional classification and gene-disease predictions. Briefings in Bioinformatics. 2018;**19**(4):575-592. DOI: 10.1093/bib/bbw139

[3] Sen GL, Blau HM. A brief history of RNAi: The silence of the genes. The FASEB Journal. 2006;**20**:1293-1299. DOI: 10.1096/fj.06-6014rev

[4] Elbashir SM, Lendeckel W, Tuschl T. RNA interference is mediated by 21- and 22-nucleotide RNAs. Genes & Development. 2001;**15**(2):188-200. Available from: www.genesdev.org/cgi/doi/10.1101/gad.862301

[5] Fuchs U, Damm-Welk C, Borkhardt A. Silencing of disease-related genes by small interfering RNAs. Current Molecular Medicine. 2004;**4**(5):507-517. DOI: 10.2174/1566524043360492

[6] Zhang Y, Zhang YF, Bryant J, Charles A, Boado RJ, Pardridge WM. Intravenous RNA interference gene therapy targeting the human epidermal growth factor receptor prolongs survival in intracranial brain cancer. Clinical Cancer Research. 2004;**10**(11):3667-3677. DOI: 10.1158/1078-0432.CCR-03-0740

[7] Chu Y, Corey DR. RNA sequencing: Platform selection, experimental design, and data interpretation. Nucleic Acid Therapeutics. 2012;**22**(4):271-274. DOI: 10.1089/nat.2012.0367

[8] Maher CA, Kumar-Sinha C, Cao X, et al. Transcriptome sequencing to detect gene fusions in cancer. Nature. 2009;**458**(7234):97-101. DOI: 10.1038/nature07638

[9] Mallik S, Mukhopadhyay A, Maulik U. RANWAR: Rank-based weighted association rule mining from gene expression and methylation data. IEEE Transactions on Nanobioscience. 2015;**14**(1):59-66. DOI: 10.1109/TNB.2014.2359494

[10] Aqil M, Naqvi AR, Mallik S, Bandyopadhyay S, Maulik U, Jameel S. The HIV Nef protein modulates cellular and exosomal miRNA profiles in human monocytic cells. Journal of Extracellular Vesicles. 2014;**3**:23129. DOI: 10.3402/jev.v3.23129

[11] Aqil M, Mallik S, Bandyopadhyay S, Maulik U, Jameel S. Transcriptomic analysis of mRNAs in human monocytic cells expressing the HIV-1 Nef protein and their exosomes. BioMed Research International. 2015;**2015**:1-10. Article Id: 492395. DOI: 10.1155/2015/492395

[12] Kaymaz BT, Kosova B. Advances in therapeutic approaches using RNA-interference as a gene silencing tool. Advanced Techniques in Biology and Medicine. 2013;**1**(2):1-9. DOI: 10.4172/atbm.1000108

[13] Hammond SM, Bernstein E, Beach D, Hannon GJ. An RNA-directed nuclease mediates post-transcriptional gene silencing in Drosophila cells. Nature. 2000;**404**:293-296. DOI: 10.1038/35005107

[14] Bartel DP. MicroRNAs: Genomics, biogenesis, mechanism, and function. Cell. 2004;**116**: 281-297. DOI: 10.1016/S0092-8674(04)00045-5

[15] Behlke MA. Progress towards *in vivo* use of siRNAs. Molecular Therapy. 2006;**13**:644-670. DOI: 10.1016/j.ymthe.2006.01.001

[16] Brummelkamp TR, Nijman SM, Dirac AM, Bernards R. Loss of the cylindromatosis tumour suppressor inhibits apoptosis by activating NF-kappaB. Nature. 2003;**424**:797-801. DOI: 10.1038/nature01811

[17] Slimane-Hadj R, Lepelletier Y, Lopez N, Garbay C, Raynaud F. Short interfering RNA (siRNA), a novel therapeutic tool acting on angiogenesis. Biochimie. 2007;**89**:1234-1244. DOI: 10.1016/j.biochi.2007.06.012

[18] Park S, Chapuis N, Tamburini J, et al. Role of the PI3K/AKT and mTOR signaling pathways in acute myeloid leukemia. Haematologica. 2010;**95**(5):819-828. DOI: 10.3324/haematol.2009.013797

[19] Zhou J, Ching YQ, Chng WJ. Aberrant nuclear factor-kappa B activity in acute myeloid leukemia: From molecular pathogenesis to therapeutic target. Oncotarget. 2015;**6**(8):5490-5500. DOI: 10.18632/oncotarget.3545

[20] Qiuwei P, Rong C, Xinyuan L, Cheng Q. A novel strategy for cancer gene therapy: RNAi. Chinese Science Bulletin. 2006;**51**(10):1145-1151. DOI: 10.1007/s11434-006-1145-x

[21] Ge Q, Filip L, Bai A, Nguyen T, Eisen HN, Chen J. Inhibition of influenza virus production in virus-infected mice by RNA interference. Proceedings of the National Academy of Sciences of the United States of America. 2004;**101**(23):8676-8681. DOI: 10.1073/pnas.0402486101

[22] Khvorova A, Reynolds A, Jayasena SD. Functional siRNAs and miRNAs exhibit strand bias. Cell. 2003;**115**(2):209-216. DOI: 10.1016/S0092-8674(03)00801-8

[23] Liu F, Song Y, Liu D. Hydrodynamics-based transfection in animals by systemic administration of plasmid DNA. Gene Therapy. 1999;**6**(7):1258-1266. DOI: 10.1038/sj.gt.3300947

[24] Sioud M, Sorensen DR. Systemic delivery of synthetic SiRNAs. Methods in Molecular Biology. 2004;**252**:515-522. DOI: 10.1385/1-59259-746-7:515

[25] Kim B, Tang Q, Biswas PS, Xu J, Schiffelers RM, Xie FY, et al. Inhibition of ocular angiogenesis by SiRNA targeting vascular endothelial growth factor pathway genes: Therapeutic strategy for herpetic stromal keratitis. The American Journal of Pathology. 2004;**165**(6):2177-2185. DOI: 10.1016/S0002-9440(10)63267-1

[26] Lorenz C, Hadwiger P, John M, Vornlocher HP, Unverzagt C. Steroid and lipid conjugates of SiRNAs to enhance cellular uptake and gene silencing in liver cells. Bioorganic & Medicinal Chemistry Letters. 2004;**14**(19):4975-4977. DOI: 10.1016/j.bmcl.2004.07.018

[27] Soutschek J, Akinc A, Bramlage B, Charisse K, Constien R, Donoghue M, et al. Therapeutic silencing of an endogenous gene by systemic administration of modified SiRNAs. Nature. 2004;**432**(7014):173-178. DOI: 10.1038/nature03121

[28] Song E, Lee SK, Wang J, Ince N, Ouyang N, Min J, et al. RNA interference targeting fas protects mice from fulminant hepatitis. Nature Medicine. 2003;**9**(3):347-351. DOI: 10.1038/nm828

[29] Jiang M, Rubbi CP, Milner J. Gel-based application of SiRNA to human epithelial cancer cells induces RNAi-dependent apoptosis. Oligonucleotides. 2004;**14**(4):239-248. DOI: 10.1089/oli.2004.14.239

[30] https://genome-cancer.ucsc.edu/proj/site/hgHeatmap/?datasetSearch=TCGA, [Accessed: 15th May, 2018]

[31] Akaneya Y, Jiang B, Tsumoto T. RNAi-induced gene silencing by local electroporation in targeting brain region. Journal of Neurophysiology. 2005;**93**(1):594-602. DOI: 10.1152/jn.00161.2004

[32] Banerjea A, Li MJ, Bauer G, Remling L, Lee NS, Rossi J, et al. Inhibition of HIV-1 by lentiviral vector-transduced SiRNAs in T lymphocytes differentiated in SCID-Hu mice and CD34+ progenitor cell-derived macrophages. Molecular Therapy. 2003;**8**(1):62-71. DOI: 10.1016/S1525-0016(03)00140-0

[33] Golzio M, Mazzolini L, Moller P, Rols MP, Teissie J. Inhibition of gene expression in mice muscle by *in vivo* electrically mediated SiRNA delivery. Gene Therapy. 2005;**12**(3):246-251. DOI: 10.1038/sj.gt.3302405

[34] Vapnik V. The Nature of Statistical Laerning Theory. 2nd ed. New York, USA: Springer; 2013. DOI: 10.1007/978-1-4757-3264-1

[35] Agrawal R, Imielinski T, and Swami A. Mining association rules between sets of items in large databases. In: Proceeding SIGMOD '93 Proceedings of the 1993 ACM SIGMOD international conference on Management of data; Washington, DC, USA. May 25–28, 1993. DOI: 10.1145/170035.170072

[36] Kim DH, Rossi JJ. Strategies for silencing human disease using RNA interference. Nature Reviews. Genetics. 2007;**8**:173-184. DOI: 10.1038/nrg2006

[37] Agrawal A, Dasaradhi PVN, Mohmmed A, Malhotra P, Bhatnagar R K, Mukherjee SK. RNA interference: Biology, mechanism, and applications. Microbiology and Molecular Biology Reviews. 2003;**67**(4):657-685. DOI: 10.1128/MMBR.67.4.657–685.200

[38] Tijsterman M, Plasterk RHA. Dicers at RISC: The mechanism of RNAi. Cell. 2004:**117**(1); 1-3. DOI: 10.1016/S0092-8674(04)00293-4

[39] Fukunaga K. Introduction to Statistical Pattern Recognition. 2nd ed. San Diego, USA: Academic Press; 2013. eBook ISBN: 9780080478654

[40] Cover TM, Thomas JA. Elements of Information Theory. 2nd ed. New York, USA: John Wiley & Sons; 2012. ISBN: 0-471-20061-1

[41] Battiti R. Using mutual information for selecting features in supervised neural net learning. IEEE Transactions on Neural Networks. 1994;**5**(4):537-550. DOI: 10.1109/72.298224

[42] Ravasz E, Somera AL, Mongru DA, et al. Hierarchical organization of modularity in metabolic networks. Science. 2002;**297**(5586):1551-1555. DOI: 10.1126/science.1073374

[43] Langfelder P, Horvath S. WGCNA: An R package for weighted correlation network analysis. BMC Bioinformatics. 2008;**9**(1):559. DOI: 10.1186/1471-2105-9-559

[44] Yip A, Horvath S. Gene network interconnectedness and the generalized topological overlap measure. BMC Bioinformatics. 2007;**8**(1):22. DOI: 10.1186/1471-2105-8-22

[45] Johnson SC. Hierarchical clustering schemes. Psychometrika. 1967;**32**(3):241-254. DOI: 10.1007/BF02289588

[46] Maulik U et al. Analyzing gene expression and methylation data profiles using StatBicRM: Statistical Biclustering-based rule mining. PLoS One. 2015;**10**(4):e0119448. DOI: 10.1371/journal.pone.0119448

[47] Wit EC, Mineo AM, Augugliaro L, Abbruzzo A. Cyclic coordinate for penalized Gaussian Graphical Models with symmetry restrictions. In: Proceeding of COMPSTAT 2014—21th International Conference on Computational Statistics; Geneva. August 19–24, 2014. Available from: http://hdl.handle.net/10447/96091

[48] Hojsgaard S, Lauritzen SL. Graphical gaussian models with edge and vertex symmetries. Journal of the Royal Statistical Society. Series B. 2008;**70**(5):1005-1027. DOI: 10.1111/j.1467-9868.2008.00666.x

[49] Bhadra T, Mallik S, Bandyopadhyay S. Identification of multi-view gene modules using mutual information based hypograph mining. IEEE Transactions on Systems, Man, and Cybernetics: Systems. 2017:1-12 (accepted). DOI: 10.1109/TSMC.2017.2726553

[50] Bandyopadhyay S, Mallik S. Integrating multiple data sources for combinatorial marker discovery: A study in tumorigenesis. IEEE/ACM Transactions on Computational Biology and Bioinformatics. 2018;**15**(2):673-687. DOI: 10.1109/TCBB.2016.2636207

[51] Mallik S, Bhadra T, Mukherji A. DTFP-growth: Dynamic threshold based FP-growth rule mining algorithm through integrating gene expression, methylation and protein-protein interaction profiles. IEEE Transactions on Nanobioscience. 2018;(99):1-10. DOI: 10.1109/TNB.2018.2803021

[52] Wit EC, Abbruzzo A. Factorial graphical models for dynamic networks. Networking Science. 2015;**3**(1):37-57. DOI: 10.1017/nws.2015.2

[53] Serra A, Fratello M, Fortino V, Raiconi G, Tagliaferri R, Greco D. MVDA: A multi-view genomic data integration methodology. BMC Bioinformatics. 2015;**16**(1):261. DOI: 10.1186/s12859-015-0680-3

[54] Holder LB, Haque MM, Skinner MK. Machine learning for epigenetics and future medical applications. Cancer Research. 2017;**12**(7):505-514. DOI: 10.1080/15592294.2017.1329068

[55] Lee SI, Celik S, Logsdon BA, et al. A machine learning approach to integrate big data for precision medicine in acute myeloid leukemia. Nature Communications. 2018;**9**(42):1-13. DOI: 10.1038/s41467-017-02465-5

[56] Chaudhary K, Poirion OB, Lu L, Garmire LX. Deep LearningBased multi-Omics integration robustly predicts survival in liver cancer. Nature Communications. 2018;**24**(6):1248-1259. DOI: 10.1158/1078-0432.CCR-17-0853

[57] Yue T, Wang H. Deep learning for genomics: A concise overview. In: Nature Communications, Book Chapter, Handbook of Deep Learning Applications. Smart Innovation, Systems and Technologies 136, Springer Nature Switzerland AG. 2019. Available from: https://arxiv.org/abs/1802.00810

[58] Chalise P, Fridley BL. Integrative clustering of multi-level 'omic data based on non-negative matrix factorization algorithm. PLoS One. 2017;**12**(5):e0176278. DOI: 10.1371/journal.pone.0176278

[59] Yang Z, Michailidis G. A non-negative matrix factorization method for detecting modules in heterogeneous omics multi-modal data. Bioinformatics. 2016;**32**(1):1-8. DOI: 10.1093/bioinformatics/btv544.

[60] Pucher BM, Zeleznik OA, Thallinger GG. Comparison and evaluation of integrative methods for the analysis of multilevel omics data: A study based on simulated and experimental cancer data. 2018. DOI: 10.1093/bib/bby027

[61] Mallik S, Bandyopadhyay S. WeCoMXP: Weighted connectivity measure integrating Co-methylation, Co-expression and protein-protein interactions for gene-module detection. IEEE/ACM Transactions on Computational Biology and Bioinformatics. 2018:1-11 (accepted). DOI: 10.1109/TCBB.2018.2868348

[62] Mallik S et al. Integrated statistical and rule-mining techniques for DNA methylation and gene expression data analysis. Journal of Artificial Intelligence and Soft Computing Research. 2013;**3**(2):101-115. DOI: 10.2478/jaiscr-2014-0008

[63] Mallik S et al. Identifying epigenetic biomarkers using maximal relevance and minimal redundancy based feature selection for multi-Omics data. IEEE Transactions on Nanobioscience. 2017;**16**(1):3-10. DOI: 10.1109/TNB.2017.2650217

[64] Sen S et al. Detecting TF-MiRNA-gene network based modules for 5hmC and 5mC brain samples: A intra- and inter-species case-study between human and rhesus. BMC Genetics. 2018;**19**(9):1-22. DOI: 10.1186/s12863-017-0574-7

[65] Mallik S, Sen S, Maulik U. IDPT: Insights into potential intrinsically disordered proteins through Transcriptomic analysis of genes for prostate carcinoma epigenetic data. Gene. 2016;**586**(1):87-96. DOI: 10.1016/j.gene.2016.03.056

[66] Singh A, Rahman R, Hasija Y. Integration of DNA methylation data and gene expression data for prostate adenocarcinoma: A proof of concept. Current Bioinformatics. 2017;**12**(999):423-430. DOI: 10.2174/1574893612666170328171106

[67] Cheng C, Worzel WP. Application of machine-learning methods to understand gene expression regulation, book chapter. In: Genetic Programming Theory and Practice XII. Springer; 2015:1-15. DOI: 10.1007/978-3-319-16030-6_1

[68] Xu X, Hoang S, Mayo MW, Bekiranov S. Application of machine learning methods to histone methylation ChIP-Seq data reveals H4R3me2 globally represses gene expression. BMC Bioinformatics. 2010;**11**:396. DOI: 10.1186/1471-2105-11-396

[69] Bandyopadhyay S, Mallik S, Mukhopadhyay A. A survey and comparative study of statistical tests for identifying differential expression from microarray data. IEEE/ACM Transactions on Computational Biology and Bioinformatics. 2013;**11**(1):95-115. DOI: 10.1109/TCBB.2013.147

[70] Xiao C, Chaovalitwongse WA. Optimization models for feature selection of decomposed nearest neighbor. IEEE Transactions on Systems, Man, and Cybernetics: Systems. 2016; **46**(2):177-184. DOI: 10.1109/TSMC.2015.2429637

[71] Bandyopadhyay S, Bhadra T, Maulik U, Mitra P. Integration of dense subgraph finding with feature clustering for unsupervised feature selection. Pattern Recognition Letters. 2014;**40**:104-112. DOI: 10.1016/j.patrec.2013.12.008

[72] Wang S, Zhu W. Sparse graph embedding unsupervised feature selection. IEEE Transactions on Systems, Man, and Cybernetics: Systems. 2016;**48**(3):329-341. DOI: 10.1109/TSMC.2016.2605132

[73] Ghasemi A, Zahediasl S. Normality tests for statistical analysis: A guide for non-statisticians. International Journal of Endocrinology and Metabolism. 2012;**10**(2):486-489. DOI: 10.5812/ijem.3505

[74] Peng H, Long F, Ding C. Feature selection based on mutual information: Criteria of max-dependency, max-relevance and min-redundancy. IEEE Transactions on Pattern Analysis and Machine Intelligence. 2005;**27**(8):1226-1238. DOI: 10.1109/TPAMI.2005.159

[75] Han J, Kamber M. Data Mining: Concepts and Techniques. 2nd ed. The Morgan Kaufmann Series in Data Management Systems; 2006. DOI: 10.1145/565117.565130

[76] Mallik S, Maulik U. MiRNA-TF-gene network analysis through ranking of biomolecules for multi-informative uterine leiomyoma dataset. Journal of Biomedical Informatics. 2015; **57**:308-319. DOI: 10.1016/j.jbi.2015.08.014

[77] Henry VJ, Bandrowski AE, Pepin AS, et al. OMICtools: An informative directory for multi-omic data analysis, Database. Oxford; 2014;**2014**:bau069. DOI: 10.1093/database/bau069

[78] Wang D, Gu J. Integrative clustering methods of multi-omics data for molecule-based cancer classifications. Quantitative Biology. 2016;**4**(1):58-67. DOI: 10.1007/s40484-016-0063-4

[79] Cao KAL, Gonzlez I, Djean S. integrOmics: An R package to unravel relationships between two omics datasets. Bioinformatics. 2009;**25**(21):2855-2856. DOI: 10.1093/bioinformatics/btp515

[80] Aagaard L, Rossi JJ. RNAi therapeutics: Principles, prospects and challenges. Advanced Drug Delivery Reviews. 2008;**59**(2–3):75-86. DOI: 10.1016/j.addr.2007.03.005

[81] Gao K, Huang L. Achieving efficient RNAi therapy: Progress and challenges. Acta Pharmaceutica Sinica B. 2013;**3**(4):213-225. DOI: 10.1016/j.apsb.2013.06.005

[82] Grimm D, Streetz KL, Jopling CL, Storm TA, Pandey K, Davis CR, et al. Fatality in mice due to oversaturation of cellular microRNA/short hairpin RNA pathways. Nature. 2006; **441**(7092):537-541. DOI: 10.1038/nature04791

[83] Fedorov Y, Anderson EM, Birmingham A, Reynolds A, Karpilow J, Robinson K, et al. Off-target effects by siRNA can induce toxic phenotype. RNA. 2006;**12**(7):1188-1196. DOI: 10.1261/rna.28106

[84] Gropman AL, Batshaw ML. Epigenetics, copy number variation, and other molecular mechanisms underlying neurodevelopmental disabilities: New insights and diagnostic approaches. Journal of Developmental & Behavioral Pediatrics. 2010;**31**(7):582-591. DOI: 10.1097/DBP.0b013e3181ee384e

[85] Bhattacharjee S, Renganaath K, Mehrotra R, Mehrotra S. Combinatorial control of gene expression. BioMed Research International. 2013;**2013**:1-11. Article Id: 407263. DOI: 10.1155/2013/407263

[86] Sharp AJ, Locke DP, Mcgrath SD, et al. Segmental duplications and copy-number variation in the human genome. The American Journal of Human Genetics. 2005;**77**(1):78-88. DOI: 10.1086/431652